The Congruent Facelift

Lawrence C.Y. Ho
Michael F. Klaassen • Kumar Mithraratne

The Congruent Facelift

A Three-dimensional View

Springer

Lawrence C.Y. Ho
Formerly Repatriation General Hospital
Concord
Sydney
New South Wales
Australia

Michael F. Klaassen
Private Practice
Auckland
New Zealand

Kumar Mithraratne
The University of Auckland
Auckland Bioengineering Institute
Auckland
New Zealand

ISBN 978-3-319-69089-6 ISBN 978-3-319-69090-2 (eBook)
https://doi.org/10.1007/978-3-319-69090-2

Library of Congress Control Number: 2017962870

Printed on acid-free paper

This Springer imprint is published by Springer Nature
The registered company is Springer International Publishing AG
The registered company address is: Gewerbestrasse 11, 6330 Cham, Switzerland

Preface

This book is a collaboration of more than 50 years of facial rejuvenative surgery, considering the three-dimensional elements of restoring youthful facial form and benchmarking this against biomechanical models of facial anatomy. Traditional approaches to the ageing human face have been based on a two-dimensional platform. The authors challenge this, based on their new concepts, which consider the human face in a three-dimensional platform with height, width and depth. The pilaster is an old term derived from the Latin *pilastrum*, describing a pillar or column, which defines spatial transition. The ageing human face can be analysed with respect to the changing dynamic of major and minor pilasters, located at key anatomical points and respected when applying surgical techniques. The pilaster of the midface/medial cheek is in fact the quintessential feature in surgical rejuvenation and the transition zone that it defines between the frontal and lateral facial planes. This zone is located on a vertical curved line descending from the lateral orbital rim. The critical principle is not to distort this youthful transition zone, but to restore it with precisely placed contour enforcement plication loops and volume augmentation with selective fat grafting.

The literature describing the evolution of facelift has been reviewed. We have significant clinical experience with our surgical technique. New research by our bioengineering colleagues, initially using anatomically accurate and biophysically based three-dimensional computational models to simulate facial expressions and lately in the dynamic evaluation of various soft tissues, offers a new tool. This potentially provides objective measurement of the anatomical changes influenced by facelift surgery. This has been motivated by the search for defining the key steps in facelift techniques and provides a guide for young plastic surgeons as well as experienced surgeons who are dissatisfied with the existing two-dimensional platform.

Sydney, NSW, Australia
Auckland, New Zealand

Lawrence C.Y. Ho
Michael F. Klaassen
Kumar Mithraratne

September 2017

Contents

History and Classical Two-Dimensional Anatomy

1

1.1 History

Eugene Hollander is popularly credited with performing the first facelift in 1901 on a Polish aristocrat in the Charite Hospital in Berlin. She had approached him asking him to lift up her sagging face as she placed her hands on the sides of her face lifting them upwards. He excised and directly sutured a 5 cm strip of skin in front of her ear. He was soon followed by other surgeons, namely, Lexer [1] in 1906, Joseph [2–4] in 1911, Passot [5] in 1919, Noel [6, 7] in 1926, Virenque [8] in 1927, Burian [9] in 1936 and Miller [10–12] in 1906, across the Atlantic Ocean in America. Most of these early surgeons used an "S"-shaped curvilinear incision in front of the ear extending into the temporal scalp/forehead superiorly and behind the ear lobes inferiorly. Skin undermining was performed before closure with a dorsal cephalic traction across the front/side changeover junction. Lexer later worked on the subcutaneous fat and weakened the facial muscles.

Joseph's well-designed skin incision and excision were correctly vectored in the lateral plane and submentum. Subcutaneous undermining was extensive, and skin excision was largely in a cephalic direction in the side plane of the face. He achieved a 3.5 cm lift with his technique shown in Fig. 1.1a–c. The before and after photographs in Fig. 1.1b, c show the excellent result in the side planes of the face, submentum and neck. He understood well that the cephalic vectored traction of the lateral planes smooths, tightens and elevates the submentum, which in turn smooths the neck. Cephalic vectored traction in the lateral planes has little effect on the droopy cheeks and downturn corners of the mouth. Vertical side plane vectored action does not have a broadening effect on the mid and lower face.

Maurice Virenque [8] with his large experience in maxillofacial surgery and a broad knowledge of anatomy emphasised the importance of plication of the aponeurotic layers of the face (panniculus carnosus) and use of suspension sutures. Figure 1.2a, b shows his technique, but no before and after photos are available.

Skoog [13, 14] introduced the subaponeurotic or sub-SMAS fascia plane in 1972. This is a relatively avascular plane but denervates the SMAS [15, 16] and platysma

L.C.Y. Ho et al., *The Congruent Facelift*,
https://doi.org/10.1007/978-3-319-69090-2_1

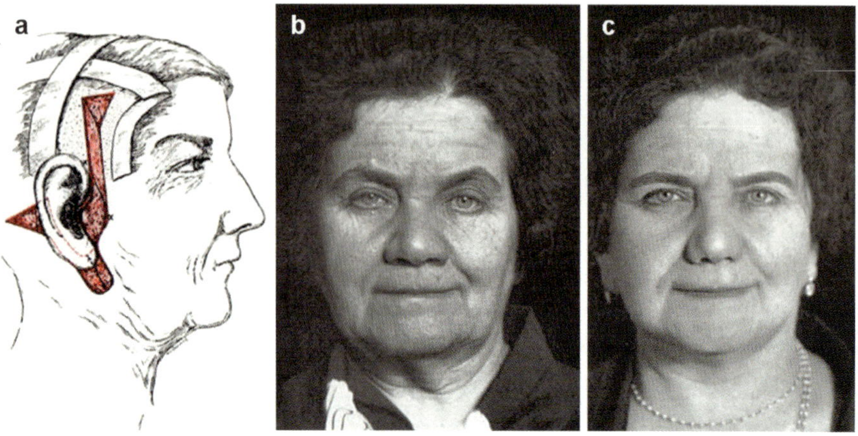

Fig. 1.1 (**a**) Joseph's post-tragal incision (**b**) before and (**c**) after (Courtesy of Riccardo Mazolla, MD, Milan)

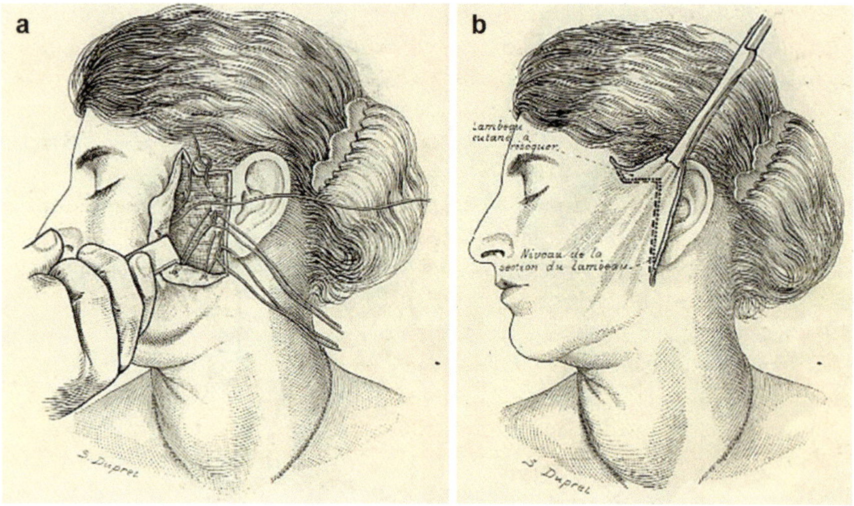

Fig. 1.2 (**a**) Aponeurotic (SMAS) loop suture (**b**) skin re-drape and excision (Courtesy of Riccardo Mazolla, MD, Milan)

which are major mimetic muscles of the face and neck. In 1994 Rees and La Trenta [17] published an extensive review of the literature concluding that most publications were inconsistent modifications of previous techniques published from 1900 to 1955 (this is also our finding on review of the literature before embarking on this book). A plethora of "SMAS plasties" appeared, tailored not to the personal needs of the patient but as personal rationale of the surgeons to address the droopy cheeks and corners of the mouth. Unfortunately, these were carried out at or near the poorly supported front/side plane changeover junction, which suffers easy deformation from various "SMAS plasties" undue tension. Hamra [18] introduced his extensive three-level composite rhytidectomy in 1992, while Mendelson [19] described his retaining ligament fixation to the skeleton in 1997. Tessier [20] introduced the subperiosteal facelift in 1979. The introduction of endoscopy techniques saw its introduction to facelift with papers from Isse [21] and Ramirez [22].

Meanwhile other surgeons looked for simpler techniques to deliver an adequate result. This saw a return to cephalic vectored correction of the vertical postural ptosis in the lateral plane of the face by Saylan [23, 24] and Tonnard and Verpaele [25, 26]. Both used suspension loops in the SMAS (panniculus carnosus). These loops look very similar to those described by Virenque in 1927.

1.2 Classical Two-Dimensional Anatomy

1.2.1 Introduction

Facelift essentially involves the skin of the face and upper neck with their composite layers of epidermis, dermis, with its subdermal plexus of vessels, subcutaneous fat (panniculus adiposis) and its superficial fascia (panniculus carnosus) now called the SMAS in the face and platysma in the neck. The subcutaneous plane is rather vascular, while the sub-SMAS plane is relatively avascular.

The muscles of mastication are in the periphery of the face (outside the true front plane of the face); they generally lie in a deeper plane and are well away from facelift dissection. The extensive mimetic muscles are superficial and generally lie centrally in the true front plane and are inserted into the skin.

Motor innervation of face muscles is usually in the deep surface but there are exceptions. Arterial supply and venous drainage are paired and run closely alongside the relevant nerves as neurovascular bundles. The sensory nerve supply of the face is from the three divisions of the trigeminal nerve, while the face/neck interphase is supplied by the upper cervical nerves. The muscles of mastication are supplied by the trigeminal nerve and the mimetic muscles by the facial nerve branches.

The face has a dual arterial supply from both the external and internal carotid arteries though predominantly from the external carotid artery. However, this dual supply has profound implications in clinical practice.

1.2.2 Muscles of the Face

The dissected face shows two groups of muscles (Fig. 1.3): an outer peripheral group and an inner or central group. Two of the four muscles of mastication (temporalis and masseter) are on view below. Their origin and insertion are bony. Motor and proprioception are supplied by the trigeminal (fifth) nerve, which enters the deep surface of the muscle. These muscles of mastication are derived from the first pharyngeal arch; the trigeminal nerve is the nerve of this arch.

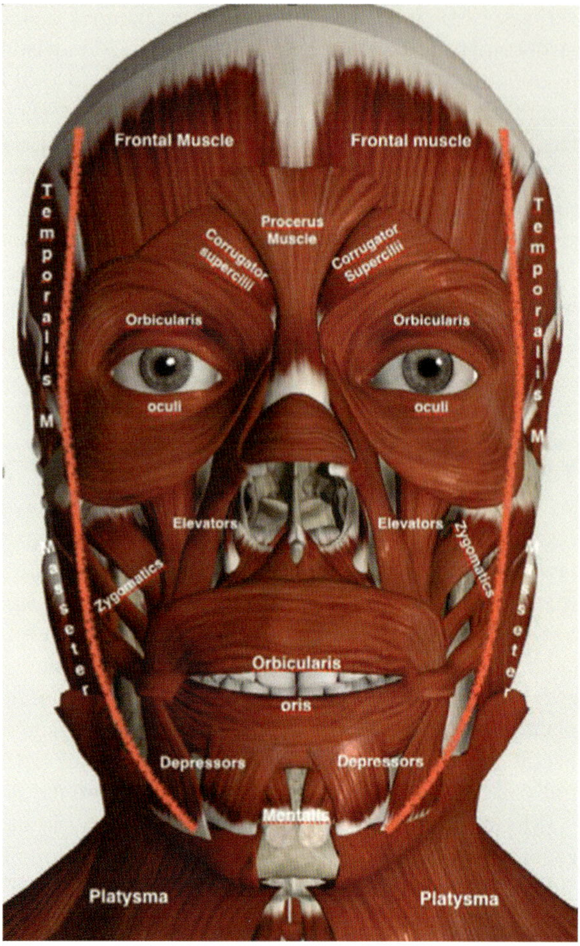

Fig. 1.3 *Curved pink line* demarcates peripheral and central (medial) group

The mimetic muscles have migrated a long way in their embryonic development and cover a large area; two muscular areas (SMAS and platysma) span three facial planes (Chap. 2). All mimetic muscles are inserted into the skin. Their origins are either the connective tissue or bone. Motor and proprioception supply is the facial nerve, the nerve of the second pharyngeal arch. Motor nerve endings innervate the deep surface with three exceptions, i.e. buccinator, levator anguli oris and mentalis. Mimetic muscles are thin and flat. They function as elevators, depressors, sphincters and dilators. Sphincter muscles in the face are the midline orbicularis oris and the paired orbicularis oculi.

The midline orbicularis oris is part of the mid- and lower face complex, which does not lie on a bony base. This large "section" (two-thirds) of the face is suspended above by the biplanar angulated support system of ligaments and septa and steadied by the "lead weights" below (Chap. 2). Apart from their mimetic functions, the elevators, angular elevators, depressors and angular depressors help hold and keep this sphincter in the optimal spatial position.

The paired orbicularis oculi are the protective sphincter around the eyes. The compressor nares, dilator nares and depressor septa muscles of the paired nostrils act to control the size of the external nares.

The paired eyebrows are a prominent facial feature in the lower forehead above the eyes; each has four mimetic muscles acting on it, namely, the frontal, orbicularis oculi, corrugator supercilii and depressor supercilii muscles. The frontal muscle arises from the epicranial aponeuroses above; its fibres are inserted into the orbicularis oculi, corrugator supercilii and the dermis of the eyebrow. It is the main elevator of the brow, while the orbicularis is the main depressor. The corrugator supercilii arises from the upper inner corner of the orbit and runs laterally and superiorly to be inserted into the dermis of the mid-eyebrow after piercing the frontal muscle. Its action depresses the eyebrow and pulls it medially generating the frown line. The small depressor supercilii depresses the medial eyebrow.

1.2.3 Platysma-SMAS-Temporoparietal Fascia [15, 16, 27]

The platysma-SMAS-superficial temporal fascia (of the temporal parietal fascia complex) runs cephalic—ventrally into the frontal muscle (Fig. 1.4a). The platysma part is robustly muscular, while the SMAS is muscular aponeurotic (hence the term "superficial muscular aponeurotic system"), and the superficial temporal fascia is thin fascia. At the crossover junction over the zygomatic arch, the SMAS is already a thin membrane tightly adherent to the underlying periosteum. Platysma arterial blood supply is primarily from the submental artery supplemented by the superior thyroids and occipital and posterior auricular arteries. Venous drainage is provided by the submental and external jugular veins. The motor and proprioception supply are from the tiny nerve fibres of the cervical and mandibular branches of the facial nerve.

SMAS arterial supply and venous drainage are provided by the transverse facial and infraorbital vessels. Motor and proprioception innervation come from tiny fibres of the underlying zygomatic and buccal branches of the facial nerve. Similarly the superficial temporal fascia is supplied by the terminal branches of the temporal branch of this nerve and the superficial temporal vessels. The wide extent of this three-plane complex is best demonstrated by Fig. 1.4b, c: front and lateral view of this complex (their action is described in Chap. 2).

1.2.4 Face Nerves and Surgical Cautions

The cutaneous sensory nerve supply is from the three divisions of the trigeminal nerve (ophthalmic, maxillary and mandibular) for the face and cervical 2 and 3 for the face/neck interphase. Most sensory nerve branches (V1 and V2) enter through the bony foramen and supply sensation to the overlying area of the skin and soft tissue.

The motor nerves of the trigeminal nerve supply the muscles of mastication (first pharyngeal arch) in the periphery of the face. They are placed deeply and enter their target muscle in their deep surface.

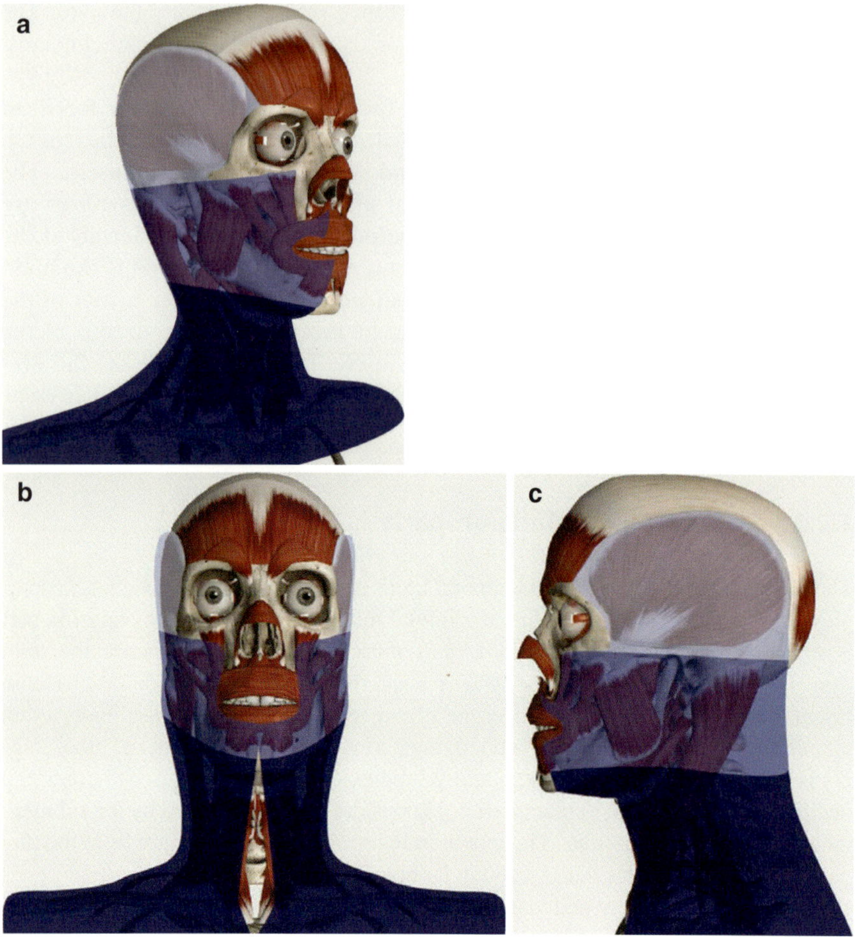

Fig. 1.4 (**a**) Transparency gradient indicates decreasing thickness of "musculous membrane". (**b**, **c**) Extent of platysma-SMAS-temporal parietal system

The facial nerve provides motor innervation for the muscles of facial expression or mimesis (second pharyngeal arch), and its sensory division supplies the sensation of taste to the mouth and anterior two-thirds of the tongue. It exits the cranium through the stylomastoid foramen. Before the main trunk enters the parotid gland, it gives off the posterior auricular nerve and branches to the posterior belly of the digastric muscle and the stylohyoid muscle. While it traverses between the superficial and deep lobes of the parotid gland, it divides into five branches, temporal, zygomatic, buccal, marginal mandibular and the cervical branches, as seen in Fig. 1.5. As they emerge from the parotid gland, they are deep, but as they run towards their target muscle, they run a more superficial course.

The temporal branch exits the upper "pole" of the parotid gland and runs obliquely superiorly and anteriorly over the zygomatic arch 2 cm in front of the meatus under the thin SMAS/superficial temporal fascia to reach the frontal muscle

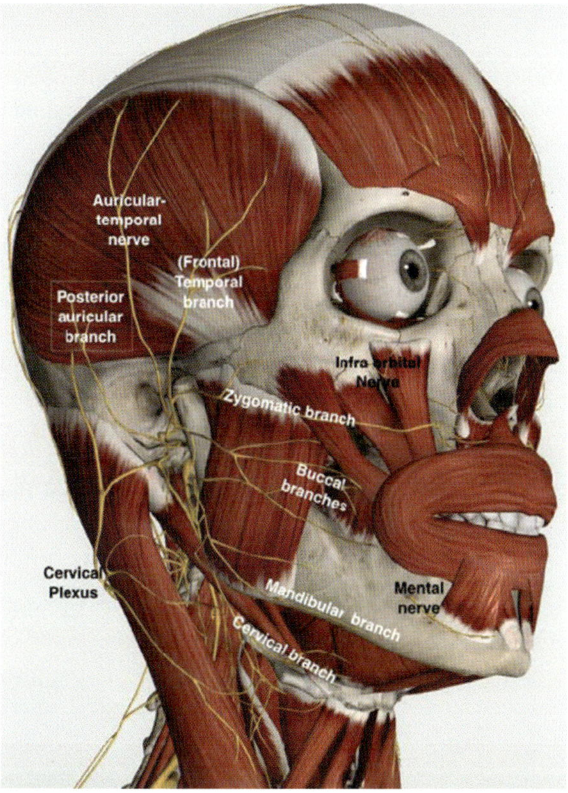

Fig. 1.5 Facial nerve branches and sensory nerves

passing close to the lateral eyebrow. These branches are vulnerable to injury at these locations.

The zygomatic branch is usually in three branches as it exits the parotid gland in its upper anterior corner. The upper branch supplies the upper orbicularis oculi and frontal muscles. The lower branches supply the lower orbicularis oculi, zygomatic muscles (passing under them), lip elevators, superomedial orbicularis, depressor supercilii, corrugator supercilii and procerus muscles.

The buccal branch (often two) emerges from the anterior border of the parotid gland and runs anterior and ventrally below and parallel to the parotid duct to supply the buccinator (on the superficial side), upper lip elevators, levator anguli oris (on the superficial side) and muscles of the nose. A second buccal branch is often present and runs above the parotid duct; both are firmly adherent to the parotidomasseteric fascia in their course to the target muscles.

The marginal mandibular nerve exits the lower part of the parotid gland and runs a variable course towards the lower lip; usually this course is above the margin of the mandible, but it can loop as far as 4 cm below it. It innervates the lower lip depressors and mentalis muscle (from its superficial side). Its variable course makes it vulnerable to injury.

The cervical branch exits from the lower part of the parotid and runs caudally deep to the platysma to supply it on the deep side.

1.2.5 Face Vessels and Cautions

The skin and soft tissue of the face has a dual blood supply from both the external and internal carotid arteries. The great bulk is supplied by the external carotid artery through its branches as seen in Fig. 1.6.

These branches are:

1. Facial artery runs deeply behind the lip elevators from near the mid-mandibular border to end up as the angular artery (its terminal branch) just medial to the inner canthus of the eye. Along the way it gives off the labial arteries and tiny branches to the lip depressors and elevators.
2. Internal maxillary artery which runs deeply and gives off the infraorbital and mental arteries exiting through similarly named foramen.
3. Transverse facial artery which runs transversely across the face below and parallel to the zygomatic arch.
4. The superficial temporal artery is the terminal branch of the external carotid artery. After crossing the zygomatic arch, it runs superficially within the superficial temporal fascia or above it. After giving off the temporal artery, it divides into the anterior and posterior temporal arteries.

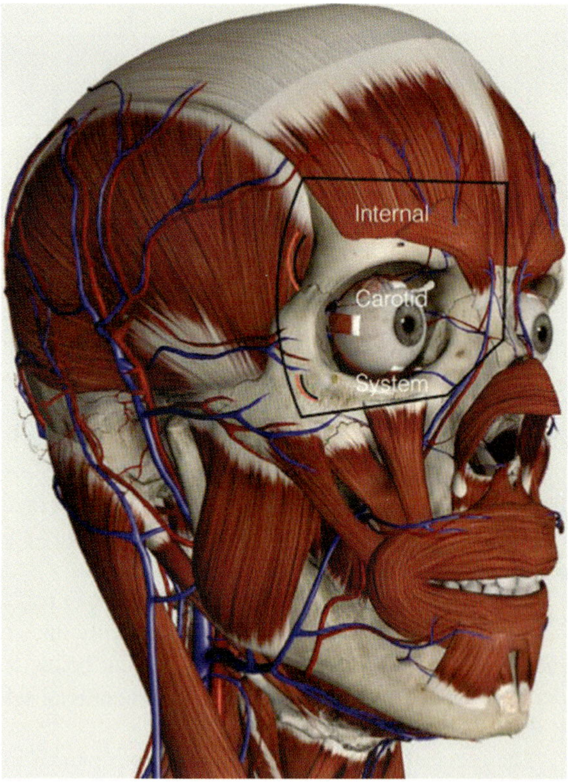

Fig. 1.6 Dual carotid arterial supply of the face skin and soft tissue

The ophthalmic artery is the first branch of the internal carotid artery. It gives off the following branches: central retinal, lacrimal, lateral palpebral, zygomaticotemporal, zygomaticofacial, muscular (ocular muscles), ciliary (long, short and anterior), supraorbital, ethmoidal (anterior and posterior), medial palpebral, supratrochlear and finally the dorsal nasal arteries.

In the watershed area between the two systems exist arterial-to-arterial anastomoses linking the two systems [28] (Fig. 1.6). Intranasally these two carotid systems coexist in a similar fashion both in the septum and lateral walls of the nose. ***In the face these arterial-to-arterial anastomoses involve the ophthalmic arteries' cutaneous branches and the adjacent and nearby external carotid artery cutaneous and muscular branches.***

Inadvertent retrograde intraarterial injection into a cutaneous ophthalmic artery branch is the cause of blindness and cerebrovascular accidents in facial filler and fat injections; similar inadvertent retrograde intraarterial injection into external carotid artery branches outside the internal carotid artery supply system of the face embolise via these anastomoses. Suitable precautions have been recommended by the senior author [29–31]. These arteries are accompanied by their paired veins. Together they run alongside nerves as neurovascular bundles (Fig. 1.7).

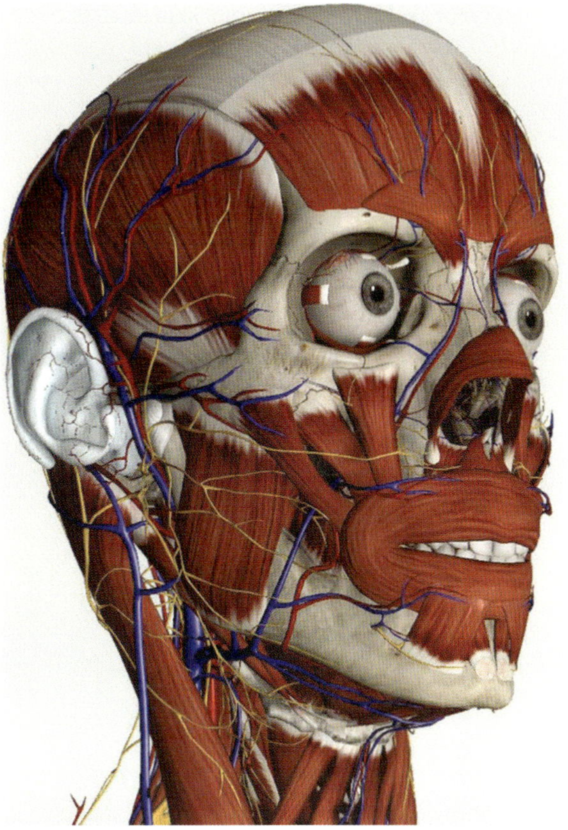

Fig. 1.7 Neurovascular bundles

1.2.5.1 Inconsistencies

The relationship between the platysma-SMAS-superficial temporal fascia complex and the facial and sensory nerve branches and blood vessels is not consistent as shown in Fig. 1.8: this, therefore, poses a trap for the unwary. This anomaly is summarised in Table 1.1.

Figure 1.9 is a diagrammatic representation of the relationship between the platysma-SMAS-temporal parietal fascia complex and its relevant vessels and motor and sensory nerves.

1.2.6 Digression

1.2.6.1 Dual Carotid System Anastomoses in the Face

Early reports of blindness and cerebrovascular accidents with filler and fat injections in the face were greeted with surprise and puzzlement in particular when injections were carried out outside the periorbit region of internal carotid area of arterial supply although these anastomoses are mentioned in a popular textbook [28]. Figure 1.10 shows the arterial to arterial anastomoses [32]. Internal carotid cutaneous branches are labelled in black, while external are in white.

Cutaneous branches of the ophthalmic branch of the internal carotid artery exit to supply the facial soft tissues and skin through bony foramina or the periphery of the orbit. Shortly after exit, they run in the subcutaneous plane. Filler and fat injections are often carried out in this plane. These branches are often inconsistent in size, route and areas of blood supply. The dorsal nasal artery is the most variable or inconsistent in its size, course and presence [33].

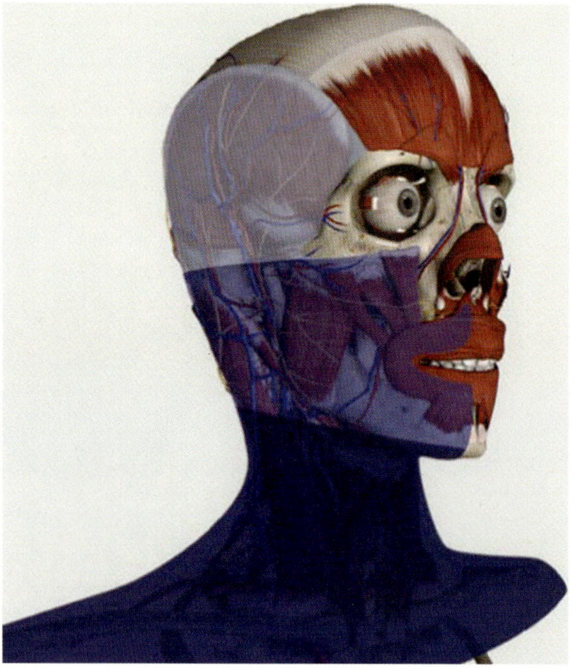

Fig. 1.8 Neurovascular relationship to membrane complex

Table 1.1 Inconsistencies

Lower face	Temporal region	Platysma
• Facial nerve branches deep to SMAS • Innervate deep surface except buccinator, levator anguli oris and mentalis • Sensory nerves and vessels deep to SMAS till terminal branches are reached	• Facial nerve branches within or above superficial temporal fascia above zygomatic arch • Sensory nerves and vessels within superficial aspect or on surface above arch	• Facial nerve branches, sensory branches and vessels deep to platysma

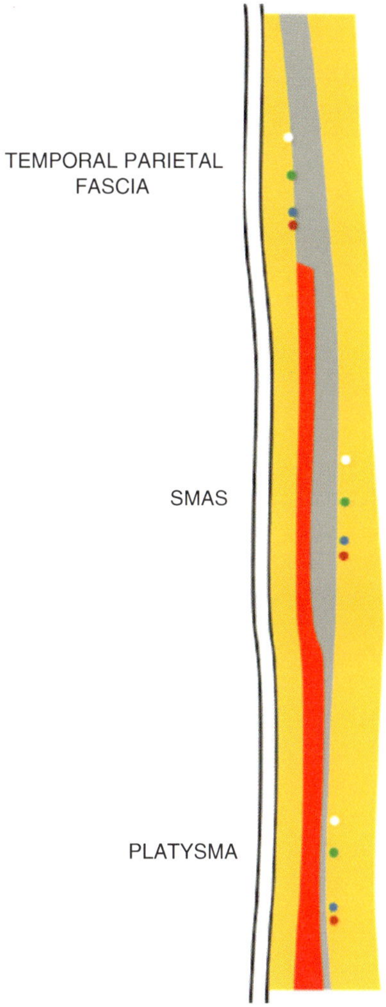

Fig. 1.9 Section from the upper neck to upper temple through the skin, subcutaneous fat (*yellow*), "musculous membrane" (*red* and *grey*) and deep fat (*yellow*). Paired vessels *red* and *blue*, facial motor nerves *green*, sensory nerves silver

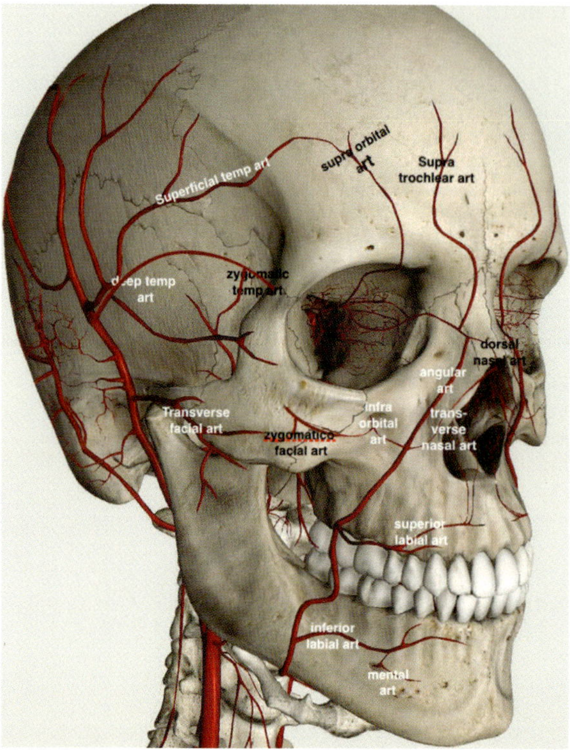

Fig. 1.10 External and internal carotid arterial supply to the face skin and soft tissue arterial anastomoses. Internal carotid branches labelled *black* and external carotid branches labelled *white*

The commonly depicted "typical" course (Fig. 1.11) of the dorsal nasal artery was seen in 34% in Tansatit et al.'s dissection of 50 cadavers; a single dorsal nasal artery was found in 14%; minute or absent dorsal nasal arteries accounted for 38%.

A review of the classic anatomy texts by Grey [28], Grant [34], Clemente [35], McMinn et al. [36] reveals little practical anatomy to guide a young plastic surgeon. Vesalius' [27] book *De humani corporis fabrica libri septem* printed in 1534 gives an early description of the SMAS/platysma/superficial temporal complex, and with it are the best diagrammatic representation of the extent and muscle fibre direction of this complex produced with wood cuts. Robert Acland's Atlas of Human Anatomy, DVD 5 [37], where dissections of fresh un-embalmed cadavers were filmed in three-dimensional views does not show the SMAS. "Anatomy of the Face and Neck" chapter by Prendergast PM [38] provides a good platform for the aesthetic plastic surgeon.

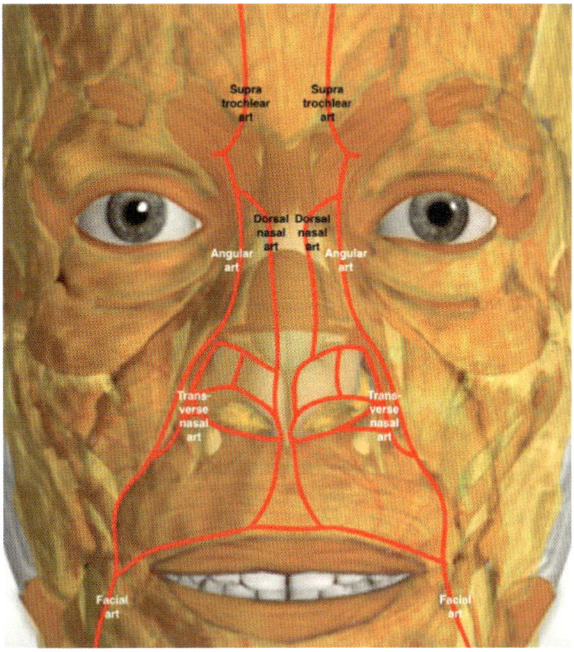

Fig. 1.11 Commonly depicted course of dorsal and lateral nasal arteries. Internal carotid origins are annotated in *black*

References

1. Lexer E (1931) Die gesamte Wiederherstellungschirurgie (Leipzig, Barth), Zugleich 2, Auflage der Wiederherstellungschirurgie, Mit 1910 Abbidungen im Text. Band 11
2. Joseph J (1921) Plastic operation on protruding cheek. Dtsch Med Wochenschr 47:287
3. Joseph J (1931) Nasenplastik und sonstige gesichs- plastik nebst einem anhang ueber mammarplastik. Curt Kabitzsch, Press, Leipzig
4. Joseph J (1987) Rhinoplasty and facial plastic surgery with a supplement on mammoplasty and other operations in the field of plastic surgery of the body. An atlas and textbook. Translation of 1931 (English translation by Stanley Milstein 1987). Columella Press, Phoenix, AR
5. Passot R (1919) La correction chirurgicale des rides du visage. Bull Acad Méd Paris 82:112
6. Noël S (1926) La chirurgic esthetique et son role social. Masson, Paris
7. Noël S (1928) La chirurgie esthetique. Thiron et Cie, Clermont Oise
8. Virenque M (1927) Traitment chirugicale des rides de la face et du cou. In: La pratique chirugicale illustree, vol 7. Doin, Paris
9. Burian F (1936) Zu Technik der Gesichthautspannung Med Welt 10:930
10. Miller CC (1907) Cosmetic surgery: the correction of featural imperfections. Oak Printing, Chicago, IL
11. Miller CC (1907) Subcutaneous section of the facial muscles to eradicate expression lines. Am J Surg 21:235

12. Miller CC (1925) Facial bands as supports to relaxed facial tissue. Ann Surg 82:603–608
13. Skoog, T; Principella sypunkter pa tekniken vid face lifting. Fifth Meeting of the Swedish Association for Plastic Surgery, Stockholm, 1972.
14. Skoog T (1974) Plastic surgery. New methods and refinements. Almqvist & Wiksel Intern, Stockholm
15. Mitz V, Peyronie M (1976) The superficial musculo-aponeurotic system (SMAS) in the parotid and cheek area. Plast Reconstr Surg 58(1):80–88
16. Sterzi G (1910) Il tessuto sottocutaneo (tela sottocuta- nea). Luigi Niccolai, Firenze
17. Rees T, La Tenta G (1994) Aesthetic plastic surgery. List of Modifications & not new techniques between. Saunders, Philadelphia, pp 1900–1954
18. Hamra ST (1992) Composite rhytidectomy. Plast Reconstr Surg 90:1
19. Mendelson BC (1997) SMAS fixation to the to the facial skeleton: rationale and results. Plast Reconstr Surg 100:1834–1842
20. Tessier P (1979) Facelifting and frontal rhytidectomy. In: Ely JF (ed) Transactions of 7th international conference on Plastic and Reconstructive Surgery, vol 393
21. Isse NG (1994) Endoscopic facial rejuvenation: endoforehead the functional lift. Case reports. Plast Reconstr Surg 18:21–29
22. Ramirez OM, Maillard GF, Mysolas A (1991) The extended subperiosteal facelift: a definitive soft-tissue remodelling for facial rejuvenation. Plast Reconstr Surg 88(2):227–238
23. Saylan Z (1999) The S-lift. Less is more. Aesth Surg Journ 19(5):406–409
24. Saylan Z (2002) Purse-string-formed plication of SMAS with zygomatic bone fixation. Plast Reconstr Surg 110(2):667–671
25. Tonnard PL, Verpaele A, Monstrey S, Van Landuyt K, Blondeel P, Hamdi M, Matton G (2002) Minimal access cranial suspension lift: a modified S lift. Plast Reconstr Surg 109(6):2074–2086
26. Tonnard PL, Verpaele A, Gaia S (2005) Optimising results from minimal access cranial suspension lifting (MACS-lift). Aesthetic Plast Surg 29(4):213–220
27. Vesalius A (2009) On the fabric of the human body, Book 11, Chapter XIII (translated by Richardson, W. F; Carman, J. B). Norman Publishing, Novato, CA, pp 167–169
28. Davies DV, Coupland RE (eds) (1967) Gray's anatomy: descriptive and applied. Longmans, London, pp 800–804
29. Ho LCY (2000) Rejuvenative facial lipomorphoplasty. Aesthetic Plast Surg 24(1):22–27
30. Ho LCY (2002) Refinements in rejuvenative facial lipomorphoplasty. Aesthetic Plast Surg 26(5):329–334
31. Ho LCY (2011) Facial optimisation. Chin J Aesthetic Plast Surg 22(11):70–75
32. Tansatit T, Apinuntrum P, Phetudom T (2017) Periorbital and intraorbital studies of the terminal branches of the ophthalmic artery for periorbital and glabellar filler placements. Aesthetic Plast Surg 41(3):678–688
33. Tansatit T, Apinuntrum P, Phetudom T (2017) Facing the worst risk: confronting the dorsal nasal artery. Implication for non-surgical procedures of nasal augmentation. Aesthetic Plast Surg 41(1):191–198
34. Grant JCB (1972) Grant's atlas of anatomy, 6th edn. The Williams and Wilkins Co., Baltimore, MD
35. Clement CD (1975) Anatomy: a regional atlas of the human body. Urban and Schwarzenberg, Berlin
36. McMinn RMH, Hutchings RT, Logan BM (1981) Color atlas of head and neck anatomy. Wolfe Medical Publications Ltd., London
37. Acland RD (2004) Human anatomy atlas 4 & 5. Lippincott Williams and Wilkins, Philadelphia
38. Prendergast PM (2012) Anatomy of the face and neck. In: Shiffman MA, Di Giuseppe A (eds) Cosmetic surgery: art and techniques. Springer, New York, pp 29–45

2 Clinical Three-Dimensional Anatomy

2.1 Introduction

The face/head is an elongated hexahedral three-dimensional anatomical structure. Five planes are on view from the front (Fig. 2.1a–c), i.e. two horizontal, two foreshortened side planes and a front plane [1–3]. The "complex" front plane is divided into upper and lower sectors by the orbits; side to side, it is segmented into two "side panels" by the midline mouth/nose complex. Unlike a regular cuboid, the face's front/side changeover junction angle is 80–85°. This changeover junction line (Fig. 2.1a–c) is not straight and vertical; it is a gently curved oblique line running from forehead temple junction above to the mandible/mental junction inferiorly with a gentle narrowing front/side changeover junction as it reaches its caudal limit.

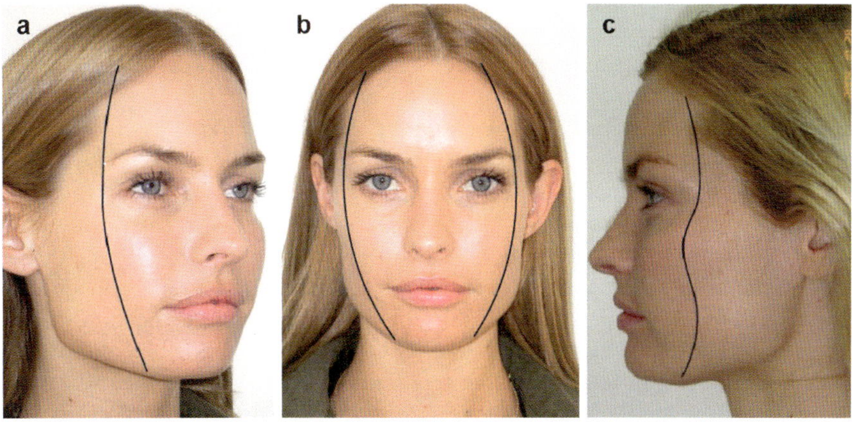

Fig. 2.1 (**a**–**c**) Major facial planes and changeover junctions

Electronic Supplementary Material The online version of this chapter (doi:10.1007/978-3-319-69090-2_2) contains supplementary material, which is available to authorized users.

L.C.Y. Ho et al., *The Congruent Facelift*,
https://doi.org/10.1007/978-3-319-69090-2_2

This 80–85° changeover junction exposes part of the side plane to direct front view. The amount on view increases caudally with decrease in front/side changeover junction angle (Figs. 2.1b and 2.2a, b); this also causes an increase in the obliqueness of the line inferiorly. This "front" plane is the "extended or greater front plane". This extended front plane exhibits highlights or pilasters at and within its perimeter (Fig. 2.2a, b); pilasters (highlights) denote a transition in spatial relationship. Within the perimeter pilaster of the extended front plane are the margin pilasters' highlights of the true front plane margin and its "landscape features".

The extended front plane shows the cheek wedge and a rhomboid feature below and lateral to the cheek. The latter is really in the side plane but is on view in the extended or greater front plane, on account of the non-90° front/side changeover angle. A prominent rhomboid feature below and lateral to the cheek gives the face a perception of depth. Tension flattening the contour of this pilaster widens the appearance of the face. This fact is significant in the design and execution of face-lifting and other aesthetic procedures of the face.

The face/head continues downwards into the cylindrical neck with its solid core wrapped with a loose skin sleeve (epidermis, dermis, fat and platysma). The anterior half of the face/head (Fig. 2.3) protrudes beyond the cephalic end of the neck cylinder. This face/neck interphase is a flattened half funnel with a splayed back. It has two obliquely inclined isosceles triangular surfaces at the sides and a wedge-shaped submental surface in front. These two meet the cylindrical neck at the level of the hyoid bone.

2.2 Facial Support System

The face consists of a skeleton base with a significant superficial fascia called the SMAS and a double internal mucosal lining in the mid- and lower face. Glands, muscles and other soft tissues are sandwiched in between (Fig. 2.4a, b). The soft tissues of the upper third and periphery lie on a rigid skeleton base. **The lower two-thirds of the face lacks a rigid bone support as is seen in Fig. 2.5a–c**.

Motor innervation of facial muscles is usually in the deep surface, but there are exceptions. Arterial supply and venous drainage are paired and run closely alongside the relevant nerves as neurovascular bundles. The sensory nerve supply of the face is from the three divisions of the trigeminal nerve, while the face/neck transition is supplied by the upper cervical nerves. The muscles of mastication are supplied by the trigeminal nerve and the mimetic muscles by the facial nerve branches.

This thick sheet of functioning tissue (Fig. 2.6a–c) is supported on each side by a biplanar angulated support system (analogous to a 'curtain rod') above. This comprises the buccal maxillary septa in the true front plane, zygomatic arch septa in the true lateral plane and the zygomatic ligament in between at the pivotal changeover junction of the front/side planes. These ligaments and septa originate in the periosteum (or deep fascia) and run through the intervening soft tissue and SMAS to be inserted into the deep dermis. The oblique front/side changeover pilaster is secured by the masseter ligament and septa originating in the

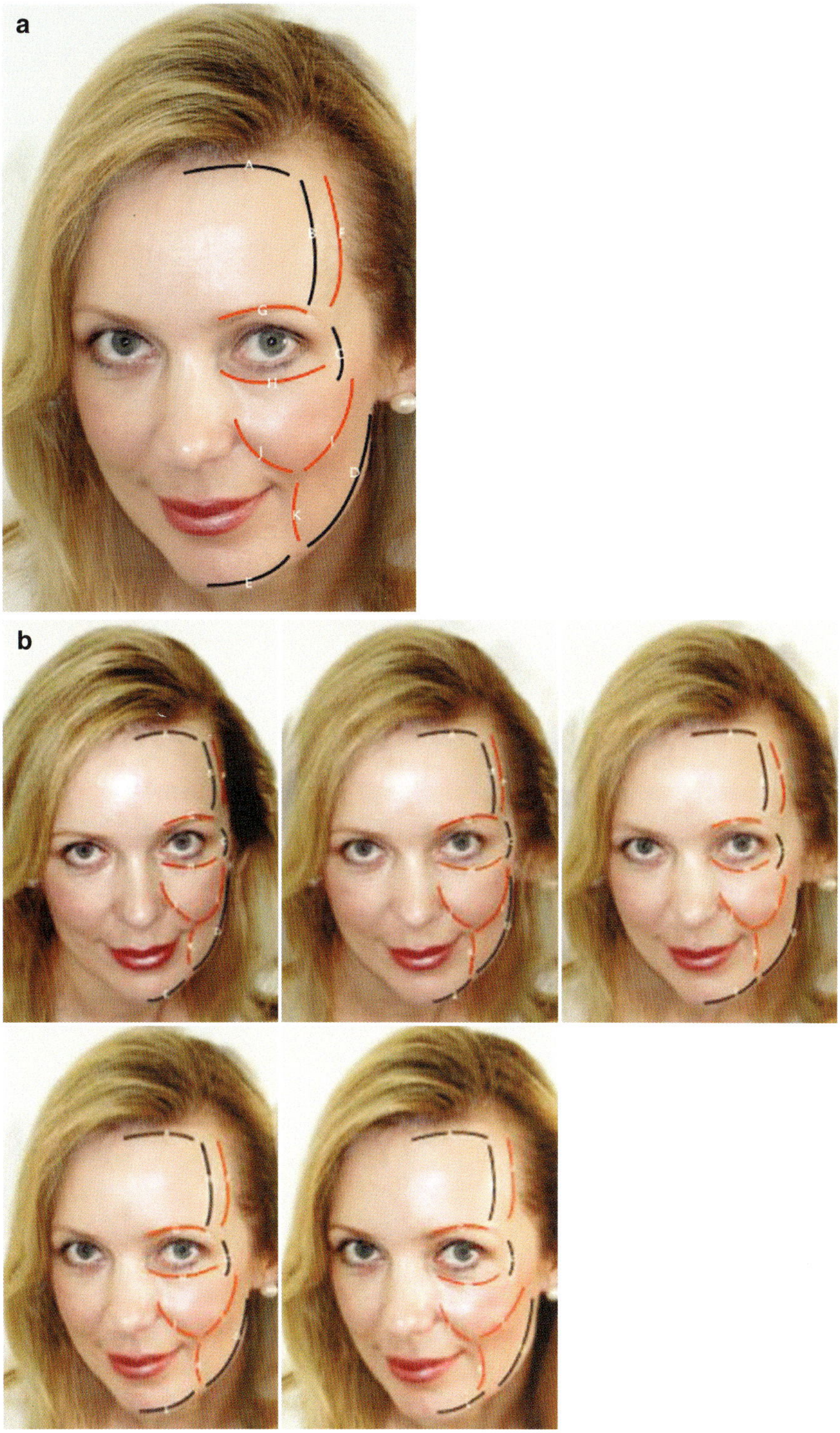

Fig. 2.2 (**a**) Facial pilasters (Video 2.1). (**b**) Facial pilasters view in rotation views

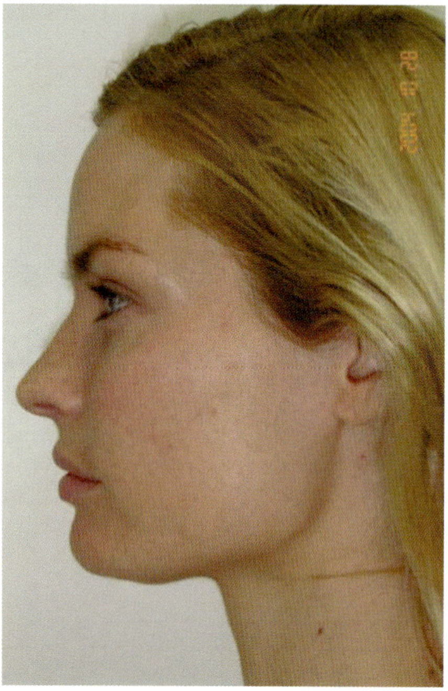

Fig. 2.3 Face-neck junction

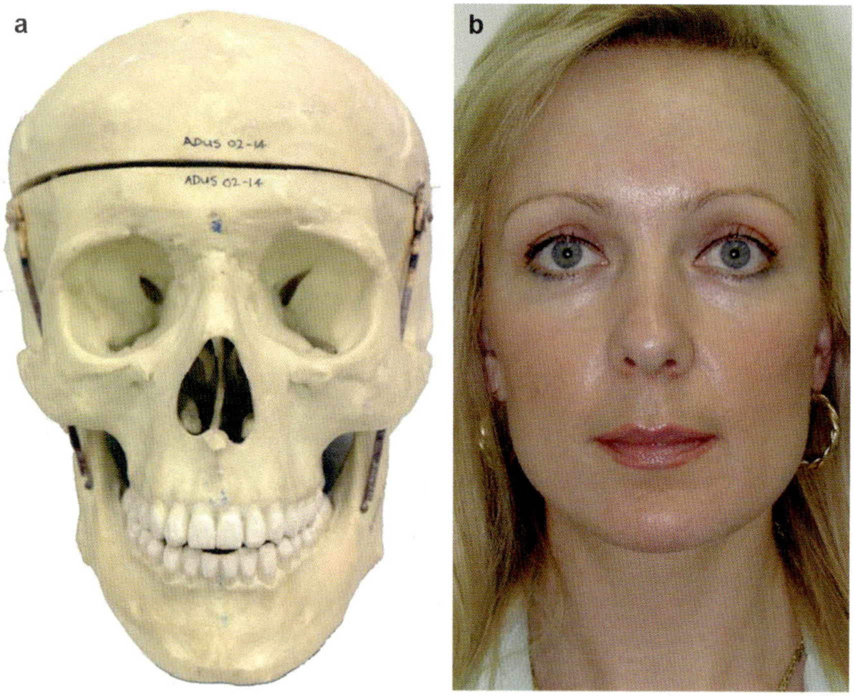

Fig. 2.4 (**a**) Anatomy: full face; (**b**) mid-/lower face has a double internal mucosal lining

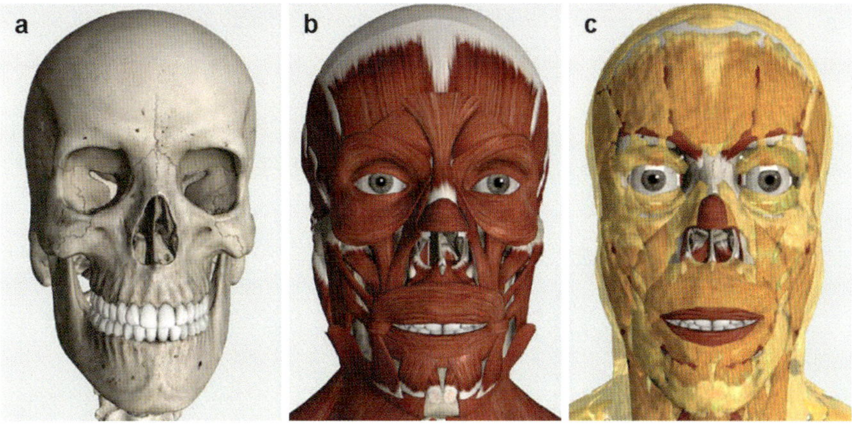

Fig. 2.5 (**a–c**) Anatomy layers and absence of bony base in the lower face for soft tissue

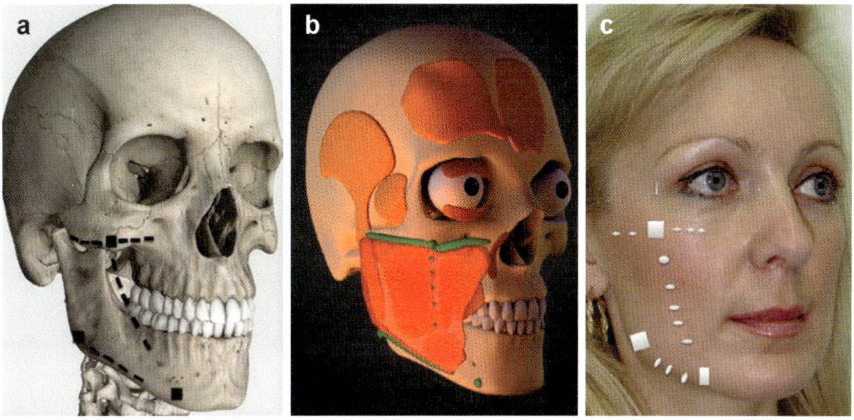

Fig. 2.6 (**a–c**) *Top* “curtain rod” medial half in true front plane, lateral half in true lateral plane, oblique line at front/side changeover junction with pivotal zygomatic ligament; *bottom* “curtain lead weight” in true lateral plane

masseteric muscle fascia (Fig. 2.6a–c). At the caudal end lying in the true lateral plane is the horizontal system of stabilising support structures analogous to ‘curtain lead weights’ comprising the mandibular ligament, septa and platysma auricular ligament. These also act as the “hanging curtain rod” (Fig. 2.6a–c) for the platysma muscle which is in continuum below.

The 80–85° angulation of this rod support system effectively places the cheek in the front plane and the rhomboid feature in the true side plane (Fig. 2.7a–f). As a result of the 80–85° not 90° turn, this rhomboid feature is prominently visible on the extended front plane. Vector-wise it has usually been treated incorrectly as in the same plane as the cheek (often with uncomplimentary postsurgical result). **When both have a similar dorsal lateral vector applied in face-lifting, tension here flattens the changeover pilaster, and the lower face takes on a broad flat appearance**.

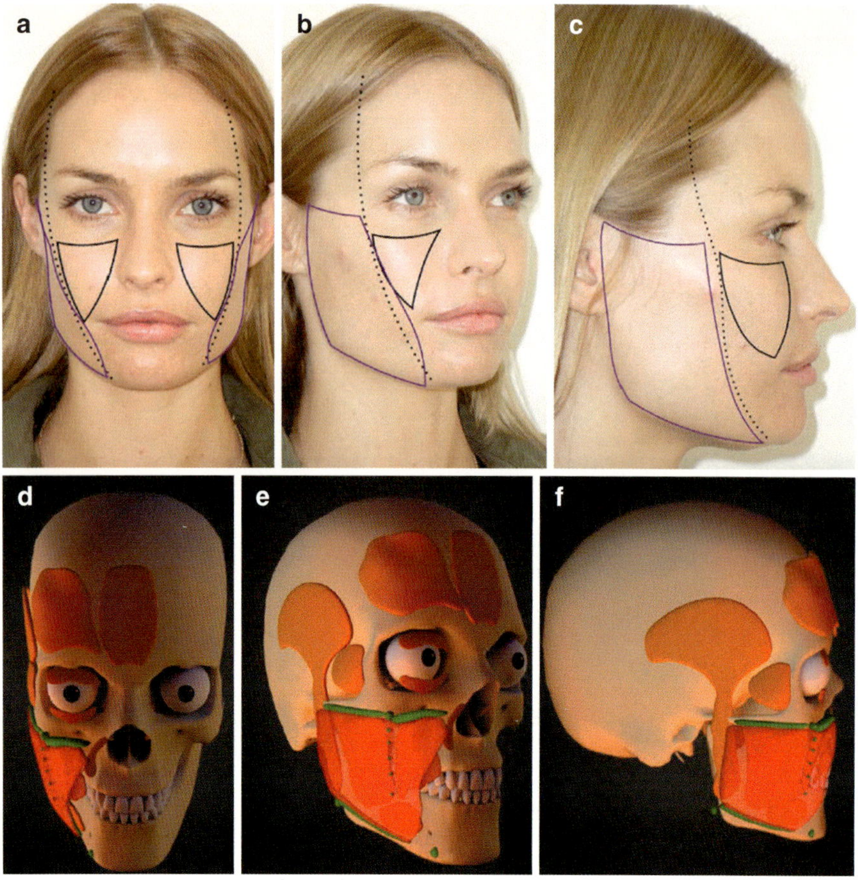

Fig. 2.7 (**a**–**c**) Rotation changed "shapes" of minor subplanes. (**d**–**f**) Rotation changed "shapes" of minor subplanes. *Red*, SMAS membrane; *Yellow*, fat compartments; *Green*, ligament/septa system

2.3 Facial Planes and Pilasters

The front of this face shows the "greater" or "extended" front plane (Fig. 2.8). This "extended front plane" [2, 3] has two adjoining minor or secondary planes on view; these are the cheek wedge and the rhomboid feature below and lateral to it although the latter is really in the true lateral plane.

These are both often treated incorrectly surgically with the same dorsal cephalic vector. The changeover junctions of both primary (major) and secondary (minor) planes appear as highlighted lines on the skin surface and have been called pilasters [1, 2]. Primary pilasters are highlights at the perimeter of primary or major facial planes; secondary or minor pilasters are changeover highlights at the boundaries of secondary or minor planes or facial features such as the eyebrows. Primary pilasters

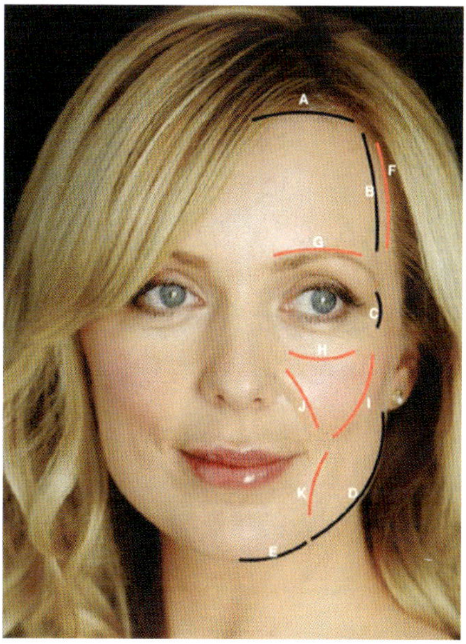

Fig. 2.8 Major and minor pilasters

are shown in black, and secondary pilasters are shown in red; they are the frontal vertex [a], frontal temporal [b], orbital-temporal-zygomatic [c], ramus [d], mental [e], temporal parietal [f], eyebrow [g], upper cheek [h], lateral cheek [i], medial cheek [j] and oro-masseteric [k]. These pilasters are skin surface highlights of the anatomical disposition of the underlying fat component construction blocks at their changeover junctions, which are "walled in" by ligament/septa suspension system.

Primary pilasters change in size, position, angle and direction with growth and ageing. These pilaster changes drive secondary changes in size, shape, configuration and relative disposition [1, 2] of the facial planes and subplanes leading to dramatic changes in the appearance of the face. Primary pilasters move centrifugally with age, while secondary pilasters undergo major movements and directional change. These changes run in tandem with progressive de-voluming and ligament/septa attenuation and lengthening.

2.4 Lower Facial Soft Tissue Composite

2.4.1 Skin and Fat Compartments

The skin is made up of several layers including: the epidermis/dermis, subcutaneous fat (panniculus adiposus) and superficial fascia of the old, now called the SMAS (panniculus carnosus). In the lower face between the SMAS and the periosteum or deep fascia is a thick layer of functioning tissue with densely packed fat in the interstitial spaces. These densely packed soft tissues are "walled" into turgid structurally volumed "compartment blocks" by tight ligaments and septa augmented with adequate

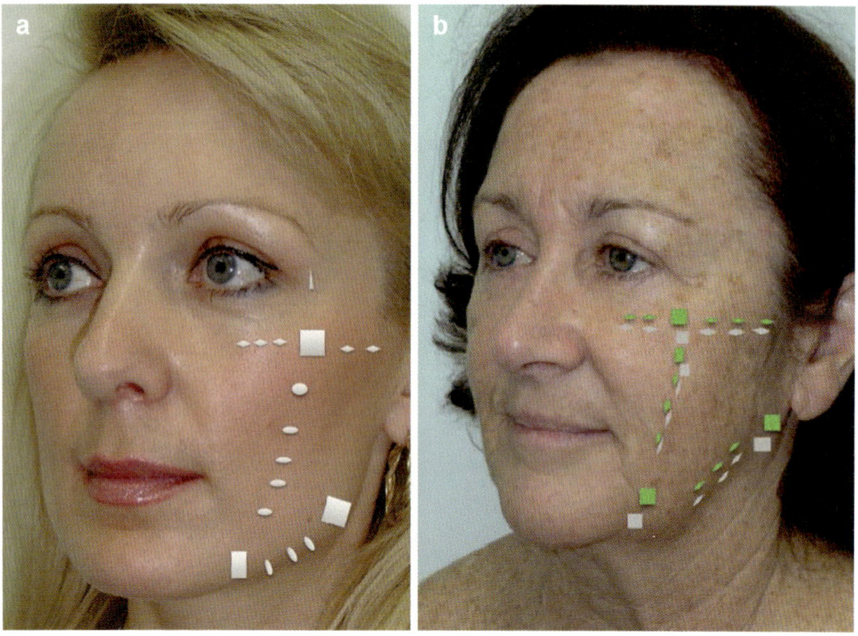

Fig. 2.9 (**a**, **b**) Ligament and septa in the young and old. (**a**) Origin and dermal insertion at same level. (**b**) *Green* origin, *grey* dermal insertion

packing fat in the young (Fig. 2.9a). This provides strong anchoring in the young keeping the soft tissue and overlying skin firm, smooth and in the young cephalic latitude in contrast to the old (Fig. 2.9b).

2.4.2 Ligaments, Septa and Compartments

Compartment decompression from age de-voluming and ligament/septa attenuation and lengthening results in their dermal insertions resting at a lower latitude than their deep origins (Fig. 2.10b). **The upper curtain rod and masseter ligament/septa system descent results in the ptotic gravitational migration of the diminished compartments along channels predetermined by the weakened existing network of ligaments and septa (Fig. 2.10a, c).**

This gravitational sagging of the compartments and overlying skin in the predetermined pattern generates synchronous changes in the size, shape, incline and robustness of the major and minor planes which in turn drives changes in the facial appearance. The downward descent also breaches the weak points in this support system generating the aged face stigmas, e.g. the marionette deformity and jowl which herniates below the anterior mandibular margin. The mandibular septa and platysma auricular ligament are strong enough to withstand this downward pressure and keep the lateral two-thirds of the mandibular margin flat and intact.

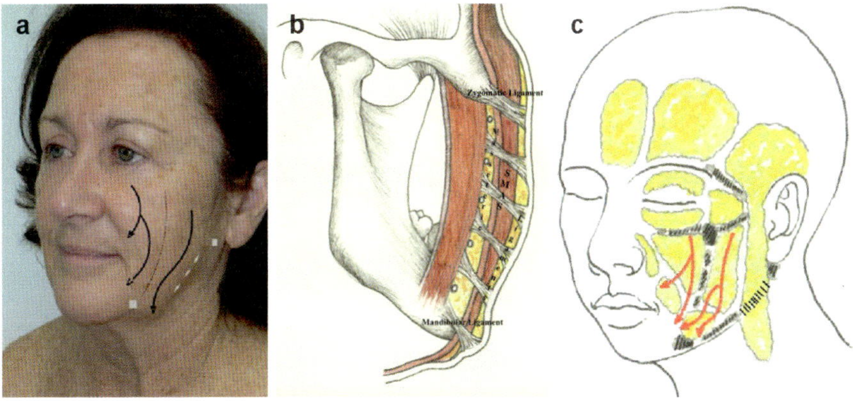

Fig. 2.10 (**a–c**) Aged "curtain rod" descent precipitates caudal gravitational migration of fat and the skin

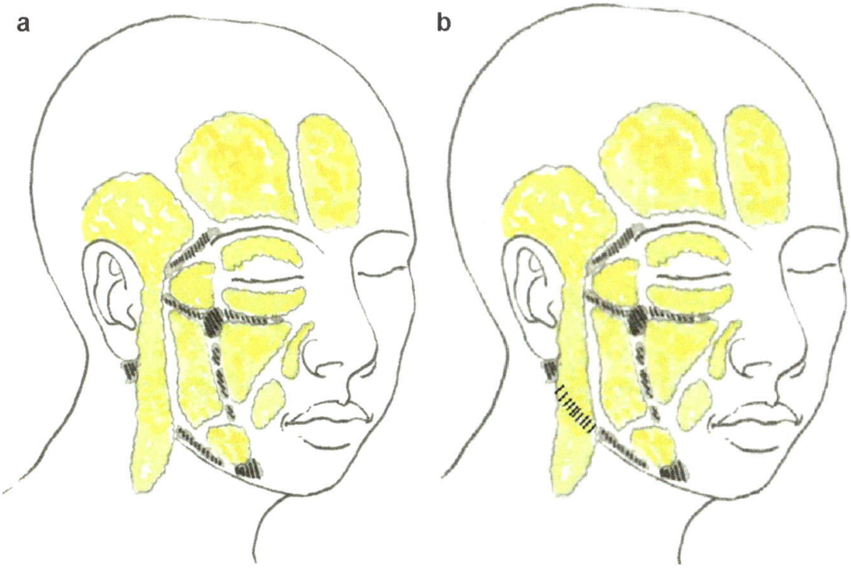

Fig. 2.11 (**a**) Fat compartments (Alghoul et al.) (**b**) Amended fat compartments (Ho et al.)

These facial ligaments and septa have been variously described over recent decades by many surgeons [4–6]; older comprehensive work has been overlooked. Alghoul et al. [7] recently reviewed these and described and named the fat compartments (Fig. 2.11a) providing an exhaustive reference list. **The systemic pattern of these ligaments and septa dermal insertions determine the size, position and incline of all major and minor pilasters which in turn drive the size, shape and disposition of the major and minor facial planes**. Brandt et al. [8] have reported on the strength and biomedical properties of the major ligaments.

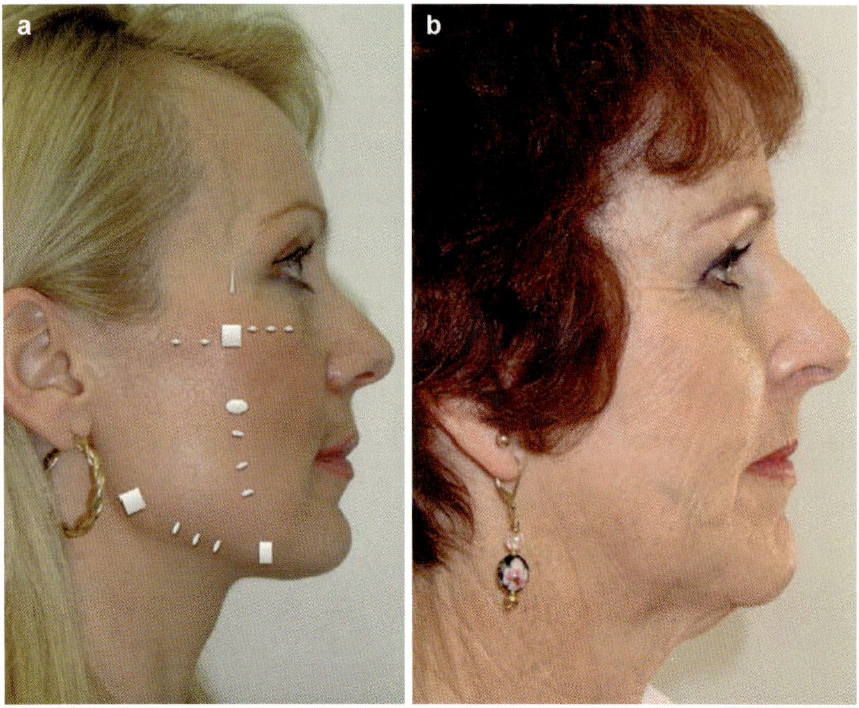

Fig. 2.12 (**a**, **b**) Ageing stigmas

In our clinical experience of treating the aged face, as seen in Fig. 2.12b, there appears lateral to the jowl a firm and oblique running belt of septae and adhesions towards the angle of the mandible. This indicates that the temporal lateral fat compartment does not extend continuously below the mandibular margin. The mid- and lower face has developed an intricate system of ligaments, septae and adhesions to secure its support in the absence of a skeletal base. Elsewhere in the face variously described connective tissue thickenings called "adhesions" in the temple and over the parotid gland have been described.

Returning to age de-voluming and ligament/septa attenuation and lengthening, where both "curtain rods" drop resulting in gravitation migration along channels predetermined by existing network of ligaments and septa descent of the bottom "lead weights" (acting at the same time as the curtain rod of the platysma) shortens the platysma. The platysma then widens (as a deformed muscle keeps its volume constant) generating the anterior platysma neck band; these bands are expression features like crow's feet and frown lines.

Weaknesses in the ligament/septa system illustrated in Fig. 2.12a generate a consistent pattern of stigma driven by weaknesses in the system (Fig. 2.12b), i.e. lower eyelid cheek sulcus, flat ptotic cheek, nasolabial fold, marionette deformity and jowl herniation. The mandibular septa, adhesions (Fig. 2.11b) and platysma auricular

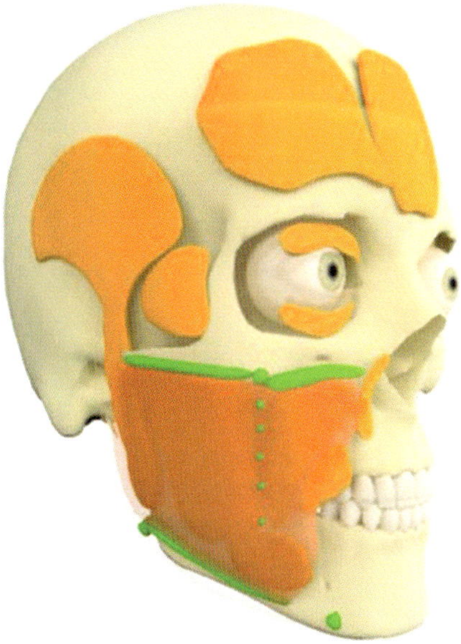

Fig. 2.13 "Curtain rod" system and fat compartments (Video 2.2)

ligament provided an adequate bulwark against gravitational migration or herniation of its above compartment below the mandibular border. This calls into question the practice of in-continuity dissection of the sub-SMAS space into the upper neck sub-platysma space.

Each compartment is a three-dimensional structure (Fig. 2.13) with a bottom which is the deep fascia or periosteum, roof which is the SMAS/dermis and side walls which are the ligament/septa system of support running from floor to roof and fibrous adhesions over the parotid gland and bone elsewhere.

The youthful mandibular margin/neck transition (Fig. 2.14) has an exquisite contour with a well-chiselled mandibular angle. These should be preserved and enhanced in facelift surgery. This issue has rarely been raised in facelift surgery.

2.4.3 SMAS/Platysma

The superficial muscular aponeurotic system was previously known as the superficial fascia of the face and is the attenuated panniculus carnosus. It was brought to the attention of plastic surgeons by Mitz and Peyronie in 1976 [9]. Many have reinvestigated this superficial fascia since named SMAS. Other work has defined this fascia and the retaining ligaments, septae and adhesions securing this membrane and the overlying dermis to the deep fascia and periosteum. Guiseppe Sterzi [10] had described this membrane and the platysma in his book on the superficial fascia of the body but has not been referenced by any of the above. He enumerated and described other muscles of the skin (panniculus carnosus) in the palm, scrotum, vulva and anal regions with their attachments to the skin.

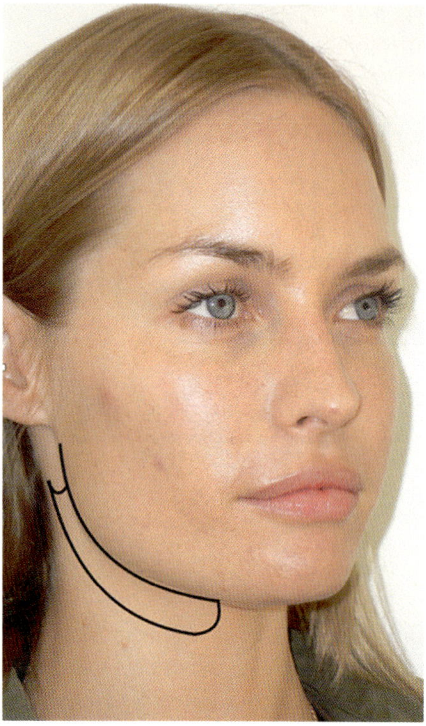

Fig. 2.14 Mandible/neck interphase

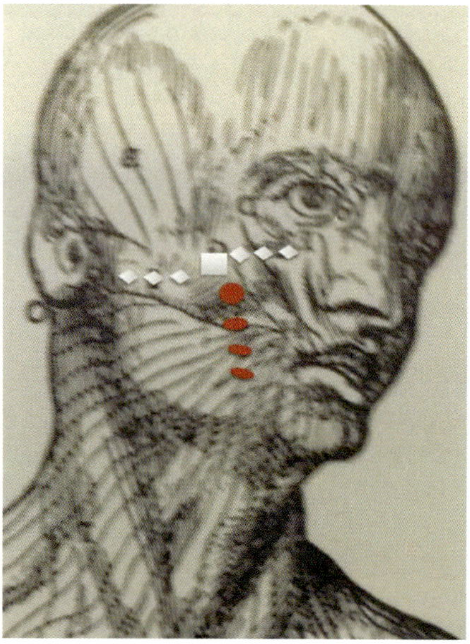

Fig. 2.15 Vesalius' drawing of the SMAS/platysma complex. Vesalius *De humani corporis fabrica libri septem* (Courtesy of Jeremy Norman & Co., Inc.)

The most comprehensive description of the anatomy and function of the platysma/SMAS complex (Fig. 2.15) is the first and belongs to Andreas Vesalius (born in Brussels, Brabant) of the University of Padua, Italy [11] **(Novato, CA, Norman Publishing 2009 ISBN 13:978-0-9304-0575-7)**. His description and drawings attest to his extraordinary powers of observation, deduction and dissection. His book *De humani corporis fabrica libri septem* published in 1534 is dedicated to the emperor Charles V [11]. The reproduction below shows the woodcut illustration of the two muscles moving the cheeks and lips.

He recognised the continuous relationship of the SMAS/platysma as one continuum structure which extended cephalic as the fascia over the temples into continuity with the frontal muscles. It was a membrane augmented with fleshy fibres for the most part and arose from the area of the cervical spine (but not the bone) and area of the scapula, acroma, clavicles and breast bone. Fibres from the breast bone and medial part of the clavicles ascend upwards to meet the opposite and in the meantime the commissure and lips. Those arising from the lateral clavicle, acroma, region of the scapula and lower cervical spine sweep obliquely upwards towards the lower face, lips and alae of the nose; he commented that some of it went far up the ears and noted that some could move their ears with them. He noted that the upper and posterior borders of this fleshy membrane were clear and distinct. He described the lower borders as wavy and irregular; parts were above, at or below the clavicle, acromia and spine of the scapula. While the fourth was most muscular, it was hard to distinguish as they came together to look as one.

This fleshy membrane drew down the cheeks and lower lips and pulled these together with the upper lip to the sides. Its action was to move all parts of the spun off face not moved by musculous substance of the forehead, nose and muscles of the eyebrow. Their action was assisted by the risers, buccinator and muscles of the lip and alae of the nose. He noticed that the membrane touched the masseter muscle and over its length to the root of the nose was more strongly attached to the bone of the cheeks [11] than elsewhere. Although he failed to note other attachments, he gave an extensive description of their nerve supply. His description is as follows (Courtesy of Jeremy Norman & Co Inc.):

> **In fact it consists merely of fleshy fibres stretched over the aforesaid membrane and accompanied by many nerve offshoots running into it from the bodies underlying the membrane; and these offshoots therefore link the membrane more firmly to the parts underlying it here than it is linked to the muscles which it covers in the rest of the body. In the first place, offshoots of these nerves run into the membrane along the whole of the neck or from the thorax to the occiput in the area where the spines of the cervical vertebrae stand. In addition, along the lengths of the spines of the scapulae and along the acromia, clavicles, top of the breast bone, tiny nerves like the slenderest of threads stretch to the membranes from the underlying muscle. All the nerve offshoots turn around and run out again along the direction of the nerve fibre, which is exceedingly various.**

It should be obvious that a sub-SMAS/platysma dissection would denervate the muscle complex and destroy this major muscle of facial expression. It would turn this "ample fleshy membrane" into an inert fibrous sheet and destroy its action which Vesalius had described as to "twist" all parts of the face not moved by the musculous substance of the forehead, nose and muscles of the eyebrow [11]. This may explain the "mummified faces" following facelift shown in popular magazines.

Recent publications of the SMAS and platysma have not touched on the nerve supply. Dissection specimens in local medical schools have been inspected. These dissected specimens (Fig. 2.16a–c) do not show the nerve supply or ligaments and septa.

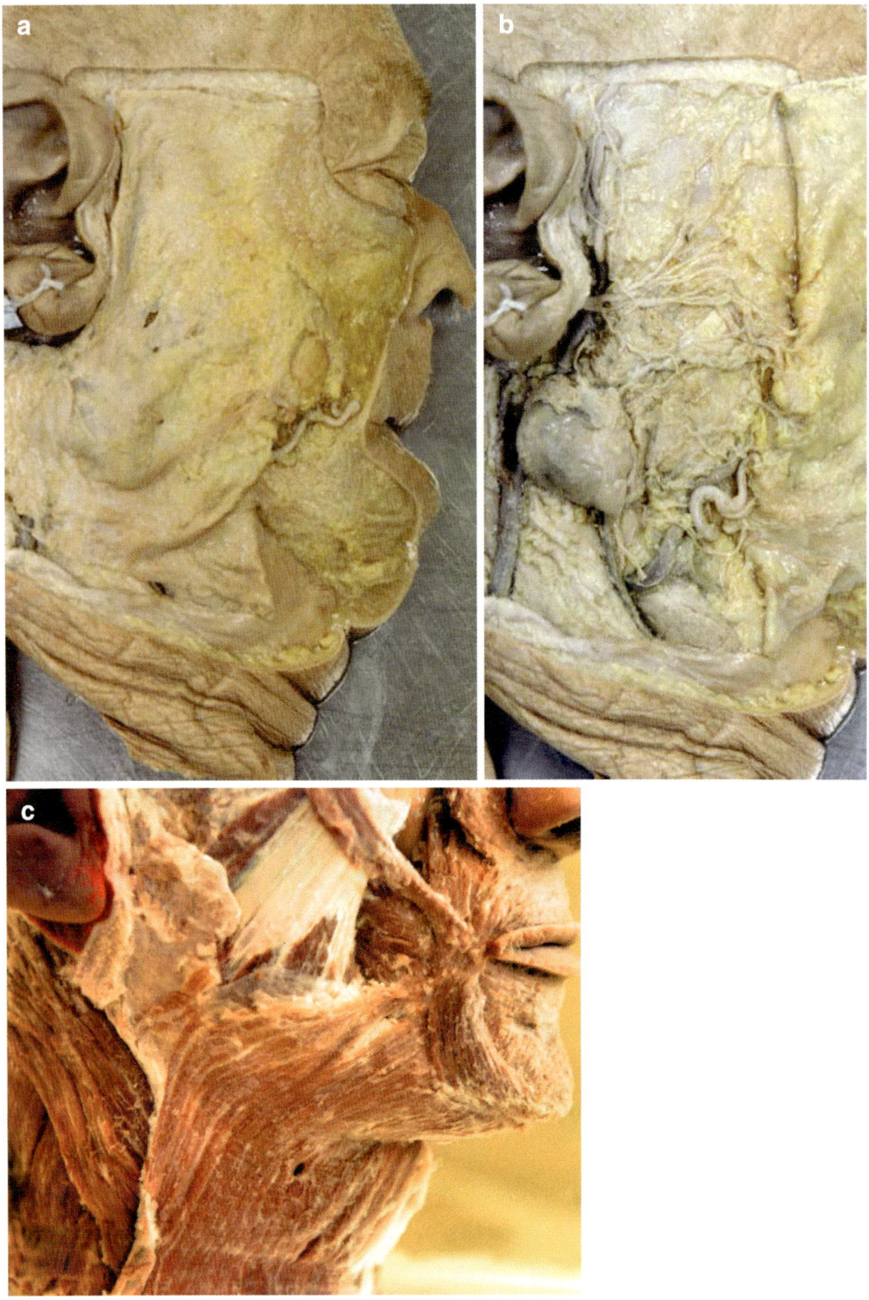

Fig. 2.16 (**a**) Dissection specimen of SMAS. (**b**) Sub-SMAS plane exposed by anterior hinged SMAS flap membranous rather than "musculous". (**c**) "Musculous" platysma

2.4.4 Three-Dimensional Anatomical Structure and Mimesis

All mimetic muscles (Fig. 2.17a–c) are inserted into the skin and are enveloped by superficial fascia with intimate connections to the skin. The bipennate buccinator muscle is the only dual-function (mimesis and mastication) mimetic muscle. The SMAS/platysma complex arises from connective tissue near the bone and spans three planes: the posterior, lateral and front planes. The remaining mimetic muscles (apart from the risorius) have their origin in the bone and are positioned within the true front plane. Contraction of mimetic muscles leads to prominent surface deformation that forms different surface expressions or mimesis. Skin and surface deformation by mimetic muscle contraction is dictated by fibre orientation within its volume. Therefore, no procedure should disturb the relative fibre orientation. All mimetic muscles are inserted at or near the front/side plane changeover pilaster; this makes them vulnerable to undue tension deforming forces in the design and execution of face-lifting and other aesthetic procedures of the face (and neck).

2.5 Surgical Cautions

Anatomical structures vulnerable in the facelift procedure are in the posterior temple above, zygomatic arch, distal cheek, mandibular border (Fig. 2.18a–c) and mid neck. The nerves at risk during facelift surgery are the frontal temporal, buccal and ramus mandibularis branches of the facial nerve and accompanying vascular vessels.

As the ramus mandibularis runs medially to innervate the lower lip muscles, it skirts just above the mandibular ligament origin; care must be exercised when inserting the rhomboid contour enforcement loop here. Care must also be exercised

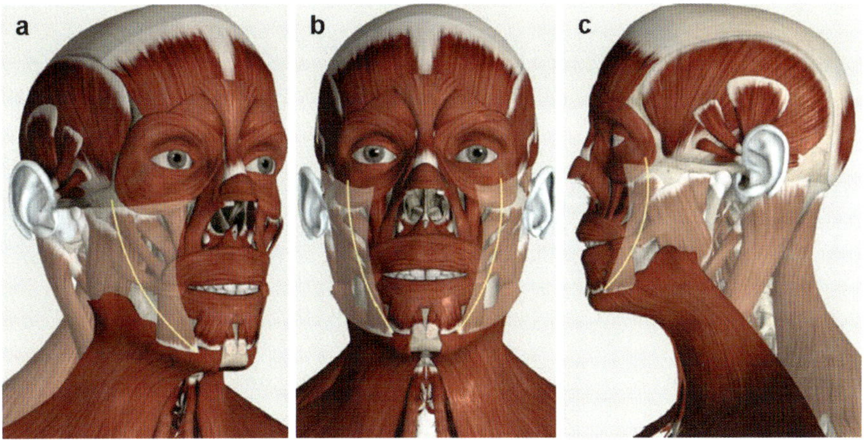

Fig. 2.17 (a–c) Mimetic muscles and front/side pilaster in three views

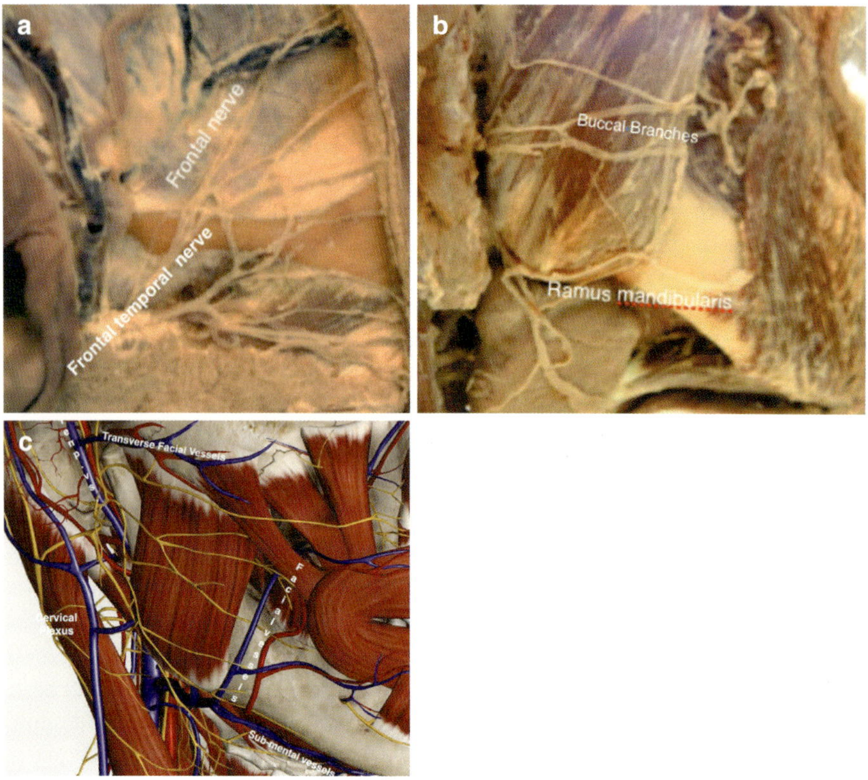

Fig. 2.18 (**a**, **b**) Vulnerable nerves in the operative procedure. (**c**) Vulnerable neurovascular bundles of the lower/mid-face

in the temple when anchoring the contour enforcement sutures and insertion of the cheek loop needle en route, in transit through the temple and zygomatic region.

Similar careful dissection and needle insertion must be exercised in the vicinity of the (accompanying) arterial venous bundles (Fig. 2.18c) as haemostasis may cause neuropraxic injury to the accompanying nerves.

The parotid duct (Fig. 2.19) emerges from the anterior border of its gland, runs anterior ventrally in the space between the SMAS and masseter muscle and turns deeply at its anterior border piercing the buccinator muscle to emerge through the oral mucosa opposite the second upper molar tooth. In its surface anatomy, it does not run on the popularly plagiarised (Grey [12]), Sinnathamby [13]) described line between the lower tragus and the mid-philtrum of the upper lip. More than 90% (Stringer [14], Hu et al. [15]) lie within 1.5 cm of the middle half of a line between the lower border of the tragus and the ipsilateral commissure.

Ageing of the face is progressive, relentless and unremitting. The resulting stigma patterns are driven by de-voluming, ligament septa attenuation and lengthening which activate upper and lower curtain rod lowering and weakening of the plane changeover junction integrity. This generates gravitational migration of fat and compartments along predetermined channels of an existing network of weakened

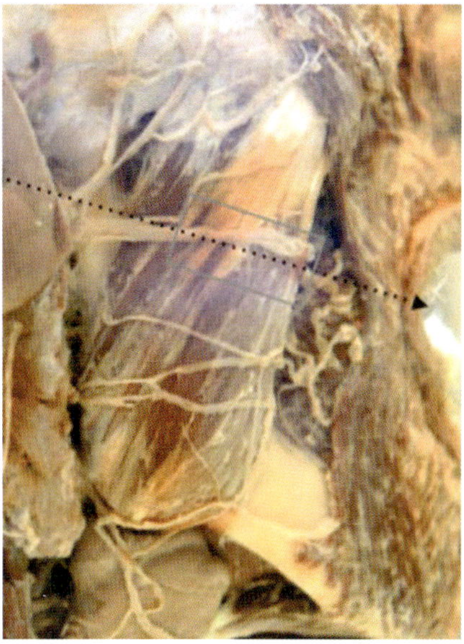

Fig. 2.19 Parotid duct and its track

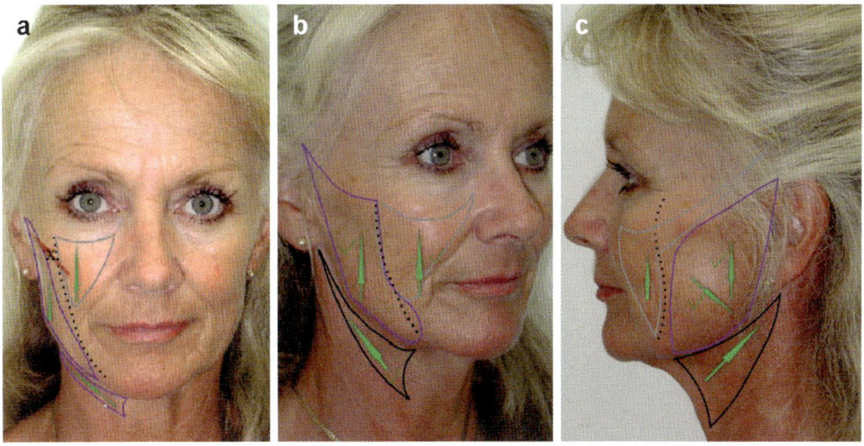

Fig. 2.20 (**a**–**c**) Congruent facelift vectors

ligaments and septa. This stigma pattern is modulated by "global" or "local" obesity and to a lesser degree facial shape.

A logical approach to "face-lifting" is a contour and vector congruent approach. The sagging "centrifugally dispersed fat compartments should be centripetalled" cephalad and repositioned at the youthful latitude and longitude of the three-dimensional face (Fig. 2.20a–c). This may be achieved with the use of contour congruent enforcement loops and repositioning the restructured facial features in the youthful latitude and longitude.

This activates a cephalic migration of coned and tightened fat compartments and skin along a re-energised existing network of ligaments and septa channels (Fig. 2.21).

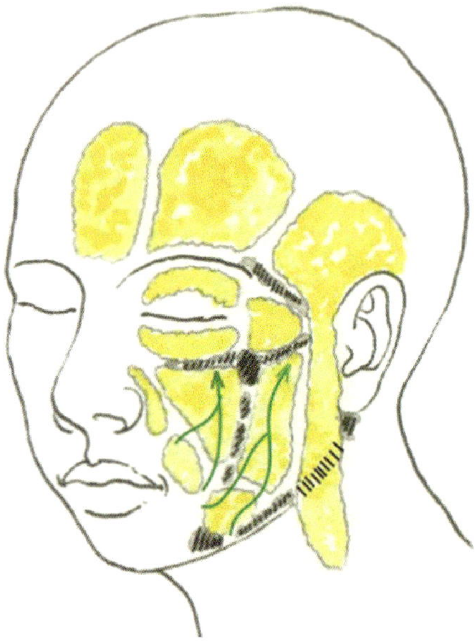

Fig. 2.21 Activation of cephalic migration of fat compartments and the skin

References

1. Ho LCY (2000) Rejuvenative facial lipomorphoplasty. Aesthetic Plast Surg 24(4):22–27
2. Ho LCY (2002) Refinements in rejuvenative facial lipomorphoplasty. Aesthetic Plast Surg 26(3):329–333
3. Ho LCY (2011) Facial optimisation. Chin J Plast Surg 22(11):70–75
4. Furnas DW (1983) The retaining ligaments of the cheek. Plast Reconstr Surg 83:11–16
5. Mendelson B (2009) Facelift anatomy. SMAS retaining ligaments and facial spaces. In: Aston SJ, Steinbeck DS, Waldon JL (eds) Aesthetic plastic surgery. Saunders Elsevier, London
6. Ozdemir R, Kilinc H, Unlu RE et al (2002) Anatomicohistologic study of the retaining ligaments of the face and use in facelift: retaining ligament correction and SMAS plication. Plast Reconstr Surg 110:1134–1149
7. Alghoul M, Codner MA (2013) Retaining ligaments of the face: review of anatomy and clinical applications. Aesthet Surg J 33(6):769–782
8. Brandt MG, Hassa A, Roth K, Wehrli B, Moore CC (2011) Biomechanical properties of the facial retaining ligaments. Arch Facial Plast Surg 14(4):289–294
9. Mitz V, Peyronie M (1976) The superficial muscular aponeurotic system (SMAS) in the parotid and cheek area. Plast Reconstr Surg 58(1):80–88
10. Sterzi G (1910) Il tessuto sottocutaneo (tela sottocuta- nea). Luigi Niccolai, Firenze
11. Richardson W, Carman JB (2009) On the fabric of the human body. Book 11 Chapter X111. Norman Publishing, Novato, CA, pp 167–169. (English translation of Vesalius, A; De humans corporis fabrica, 1543 Bale)
12. Grey H (1858) The anatomy: descriptive and surgical. John W. Parker & Son, London, p 593
13. Sinnathamby CS (2011) Last's anatomy: regional and applied. Churchill Livingstone, Elsevier, Edinburgh, p 277
14. Stringer MD, Mirjalili SA, Meredith SJ, Muirhead JC (2012) Redefining the surface anatomy of the parotid duct: an in vivo ultrasound study. Plast Reconstr Surg 130(5):1032–1037
15. Hu KS, Kim ST, Hur MS, Park JH, Song WC, Koh KS, Kim HJ (2010) Topography of the master muscle in relation to treatment with botulinum toxin type A. Oral Surg Oral Med Oral Pathol Oral Radiol 110(2):167–171

Biomechanics of Three-Dimensional Face 3

3.1 Introduction

As stated in the preceding chapters, the human head is a three-dimensional, structurally as well as functionally complex unit that consists of several anatomical structures. These include bones, muscles, fat, ligaments, skin and vessels. It contains delicate expressive areas while the rest of the head is relatively immobile and contributes virtually nothing to the formation of facial expressions and gestures. There exist over 60 muscles in the face; most are bilateral muscles (exist in pairs), for serving different day-to-day functions such as mastication, vision and communication.

Facial movements are generated by coordinated actions of over 40 muscles in the face [1]. The muscles responsible for facial expressions are known as mimetic muscles [2] and innervated by the facial nerve (cranial nerve VII). These muscles are mostly situated in the superficial soft tissue region of the face [3]. The masseter and buccinator muscles are exceptions as they occupy both deep and superficial regions. The former functions primarily as a masticatory muscle, while the latter plays a dual role as a masticatory as well as mimetic muscle. As such, the buccinator's fascicular organisation is bipennate (more details on pennation later). Upon contraction, the superficial region slides over the deep tissue region (both soft and hard) causing substantial movement of the skin. This results in visible changes in facial appearances (e.g. wrinkling, raising of mouth corners, etc.) for communication and expressing emotions. Figure 3.1 depicts the organisation of tissue structures in the human face.

Organisation of soft tissue structures in the human face is complex, and these structures have distinct constitutive (mechanical) properties. Based on their constitutive properties, three main groups of soft tissue structures can be identified. They are the skin, subcutaneous fat and muscles. From mechanical strength point of view, the skin that consists of several sub-layers is the stiffest, while the subcutaneous fat

Electronic Supplementary Material The online version of this chapter (doi:10.1007/978-3-319-69090-2_3) contains supplementary material, which is available to authorized users.

L.C.Y. Ho et al., *The Congruent Facelift*,
https://doi.org/10.1007/978-3-319-69090-2_3

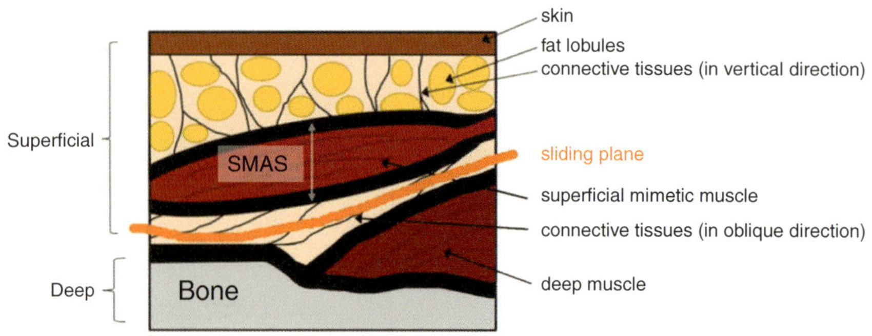

Fig. 3.1 Organisation of tissues in the human face. Superficial layer consists of the skin, subcutaneous fat and mimetic muscles, and the deep layer consists of deep muscles and bones (*Adapted from Hung et al.* [1])

offers the least resistance to deformation. From biomechanical point of view, both structure and function of these tissues play an important role. In this chapter, the focus will be primarily on the biomechanical characteristics of soft tissues, in particular mimetic muscles and the face as a whole.

3.2 Mechanics of Mimetic Muscles

Mechanics of biological structures, either soft or hard, is governed by the same engineering principles applicable to other engineering structures (e.g. reinforced concrete beams, steel columns). Thus, any analysis involving mechanics of deformation of a tissue structure needs to include the following.

1. Firstly, pertinent governing equations are necessary to describe the physics of the problem. These are based on laws of conservation, namely, mass, momentum and energy. For solids that undergo isothermal (constant temperature) deformations, only momentum equation is required. Conservation of mass is automatically satisfied for solids, and there is no energy change due to constant temperature conditions. Thus, any deformed state, intermediate or final, of the muscle (tissue) structure must satisfy physics described by the momentum equation all the time.
2. Secondly, relationship between displacement and strain must be established. This is known as kinematics associated with deformation. The displacement is the distance between a point in the body before and after deformation in three dimensions, while the strain is a measure of deformation.
3. Thirdly, knowledge of the constitution of the tissue material is required. This is described using a stress-strain or in simple terms load-deformation relationship. This information is usually obtained from experiments conducted under controlled conditions. Thus, any deformation (strain) at a given point of the solid body (tissue) must satisfy the experimentally measured load (stress).

4. Fourthly, in order to close the problem mathematically or simply to ensure that there are enough equations to solve the unknown variables, suitable boundary conditions must be prescribed. In the case of biological structures, these are usually physiologically realistic boundary conditions. For instance, when a muscle attaches to a rigid bony structure, it is prescribed as a displacement or Dirichlet boundary condition.
5. Finally, constraints, which are encountered in any practical problem irrespective of whether the problem at hand is to deal with an engineering or a biological structure, must be imposed. In the case of muscles, two types of constraints are of interest: (a) isochoric or constant volume constraints and (b) prevention of interpenetration of solid tissue structures.

The above will be discussed next in relation to muscles in general without referring to a specific muscle type such as mimetic muscles. In order to simplify the mathematics involved in the following discussion, a one-dimensional muscle is considered. In one-dimensional case, only scalar variables are required as opposed to vector and tensor variables in higher dimensional analysis.

Governing Equations
Although formulation of a dynamic deformation problem is not cumbersome, usually soft tissue deformation analysis is performed using quasi-static formulation. In this approach, the inertial force due to acceleration of deformable solid body is neglected. In other words, the overall deformation is described using a series of static incremental deformations. The one-dimensional or the scalar form of the momentum equation that describes the static equilibrium of the body can be written as

$$\frac{\partial \sigma}{\partial x} + b = 0$$

where σ is the Cauchy stress, b represents body forces such as gravity and x is the spatial location of the point in solid continuum. This equation is called Cauchy's equation to honour Augustine Cauchy, a French physicist/mathematician, who developed the equation by applying the Newton's second law of motion to deformable solids. Although σ is a scalar variable in one dimension, it is a tensor variable with nine components in three dimensions. The above equation deals with equilibrium associated with the translational motion hence often called linear momentum equation. Strictly speaking, it is necessary to consider not only translational but rotational equilibrium as well. If rotational equilibrium of the deformable solid is considered, the Cauchy stress tensor in three dimensions with nine components will reduce to a symmetric tensor.

Kinematics of Deformation
The strain, which is a measure of deformation as stated in the preceding section, is a function of displacement gradient. Mathematically this function can be written as

$$e = \frac{\partial u}{\partial x} + \frac{1}{2}\left(\frac{\partial u}{\partial x}\right)^2$$

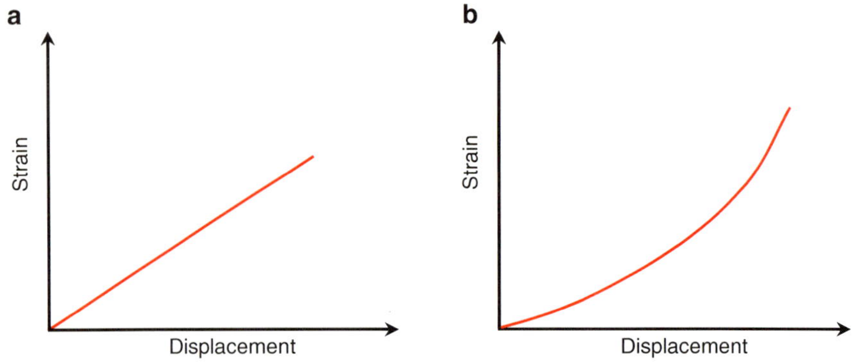

Fig. 3.2 Displacement-strain. (**a**) Linear relationship leading to a kinematically linear deformation. (**b**) Non-linear relationship as found in muscle deformation leading to finite or kinematically non-linear deformation

where e is the strain, u is the displacement and x is again the spatial location. The term $\partial u/\partial x$ is called the displacement gradient. For kinematically small deformations, such as those found in engineering solid bodies, the quadratic term can be neglected, and the strain becomes a linear function of the displacement gradient. These are called kinematically linear deformations. However, soft tissues such as muscles often undergo relatively larger deformations, and therefore the quadratic term cannot be simply dropped. As such, strain becomes a non-linear function of the displacement gradient and is termed non-linear or finite strain (Fig. 3.2).

Constitutive Properties

When a deformable solid is subject to loading, intermolecular forces will be induced, and the ensuing deformation is controlled by these internal forces. These are passive resistive forces, and the stress that was mentioned in the preceding section represents these internal forces/loadings. Note that stress is force per unit area, and hence it can be considered as passive force intensity. Every deformable solid has a unique relationship between the amount of deformation (strain) and force that causes it, which can be described using stress. However, this relationship must be experimentally determined, and the data so obtained are fitted to define the "constitutive model" of the material (tissue). This essentially tells how much stress is induced for a given strain. The stress so determined will be used in momentum equation. Furthermore, the stress-strain relationship of a solid can be linear or non-linear. Most engineering materials, such as steel or concrete, exhibit linear constitutive properties over the range of interest. On the other hand, most biological soft tissues (e.g. muscles) show non-linear characteristics.

The stress-strain relationship of muscles is structure dependent. In particular, constitutive properties along the fibre or fascicular direction (will be discussed in detail under structure section below) are different to those in other directions. The tissues that have a preferential direction such as muscles are called transversely isotropic materials. Rubber, on the other hand, does not possess any preferential direction and is called an isotropic material. Cardiac muscle tissue properties can be defined with respect to three mutually orthogonal directions, and hence it is called an orthotropic

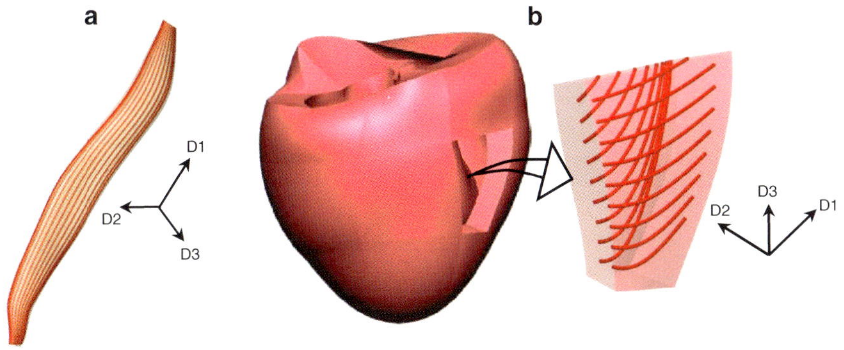

Fig. 3.3 Structure-based mutually orthogonal directions for defining constitutive properties. (**a**) Transversely isotropic skeletal/mimetic muscle—D1 is along the fibre direction and has different properties to D2 and D3, while the properties in the latter two directions are identical. (**b**) Orthotropic cardiac muscle—properties in all three directions are different, D1 is along the fibre, D2 represents sheet direction where fibres lie and D3 is normal to sheets

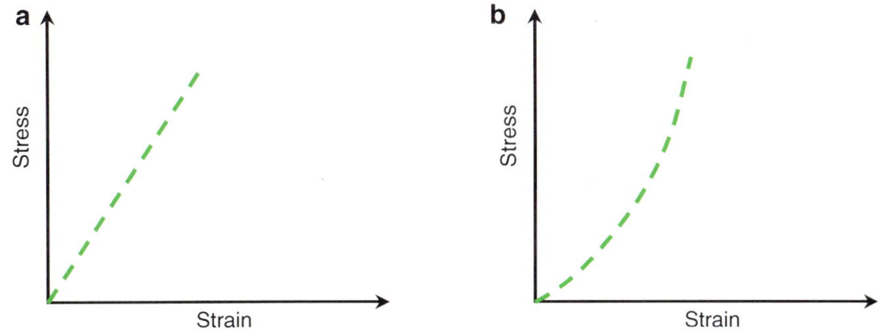

Fig. 3.4 Constitutive (stress-strain) behaviour of deformable solids. (**a**) Linear and (**b**) non-linear material

tissue. These directions are defined with respect to the structural organisation of the tissue. In muscles, principal direction is defined along the fibre direction, and two more mutually orthogonal directions orthogonal to the fibre direction are defined to form a three-dimensional coordinate system (Fig. 3.3). For instance, cardiac muscle is a highly non-linear tissue [4] meaning there is exponential increase in stress as strain increases or in simple terms, the more the body deforms the larger the force is required to maintain the deformation (Fig. 3.4).

Boundary Conditions

In deformable body solid mechanics, three types of boundary conditions are encountered. The first type of boundary condition is known as the displacement or Dirichlet boundary conditions. With these, it is possible to prescribe a spatial location of a point or points on the solid surface. Once a spatial location is prescribed, the point simply assumes the location and does not have to satisfy governing equations or constitutive relationship. These are the predominantly used boundary conditions in

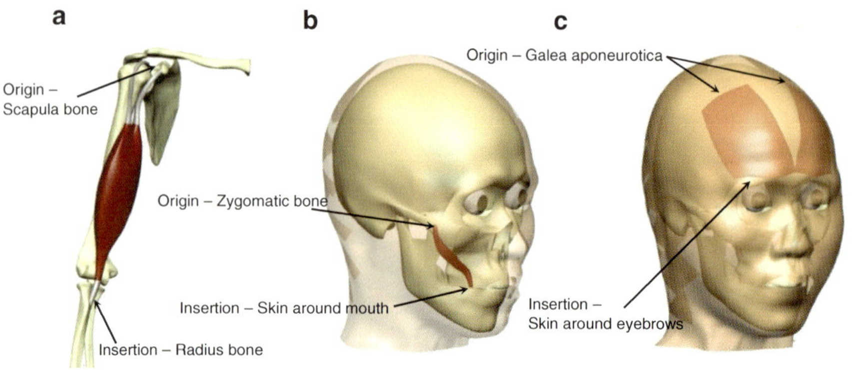

Fig. 3.5 Muscle attachments. (**a**) Skeletal muscle, biceps brachii; (**b**) mimetic muscle, zygomaticus major; (**c**) mimetic muscle, frontalis

muscles. They can be used to prescribe muscle attachments on rigid bony structures (Fig. 3.5a). Note that if a muscle inserts into a soft tissue (e.g. zygomaticus major; more details on mimetic muscle attachments in Sect. 3.2.1), the displacement boundary conditions cannot be used at the insertion point.

The second type of boundary conditions is called the force or Neumann boundary conditions. These are used to prescribe a point or distributed force/load acting on the surface of a solid structure. This type of boundary conditions is rarely used in muscle mechanics unless there is external force acting on the muscle surface (Fig. 3.4b). The third type of boundary conditions is known as the Robin boundary conditions. These are formulated as a combination of the first two types (i.e. Dirichlet and Neumann). Although the contact between solid bodies can be put into this category, it (contact interactions) can be better described under constraints. Note that in muscle mechanics, it is important to consider contact interaction between various types of tissue structures and these are usually dealt with by imposing suitable constraints.

Constraints

It was stated in the preceding paragraph, constraints are an integral part of tissue mechanics. As far as muscle or soft tissue mechanics is concerned, there are two constraints of importance. Firstly, it is well documented that striated muscles (more details in Sect. 3.2.1) preserve their volumes. Experimentally observed volume changes during deformation (contraction) of muscles have been reported insignificant. Any changes in muscle volume will very rapidly (within milliseconds) diminish, and the muscle will assume its original volume irrespective to the shape [5]. As such, it is required to impose this constraint implicitly to ensure that the predicted shape upon muscle activation is physiologically correct. The second constraint that needs to be imposed is to ensure that there is no interpenetration between adjacent tissue structures. This constraint is an obvious phenomenon as it is impossible to have interpenetration between two or more solid bodies, rigid or complaint.

3.2.1 Mimetic Muscles

There are three types of striated muscles found in the human body, namely, skeletal, mimetic and cardiac muscle. Striated muscles have visible bands under a microscope. Of the three, the first two types contract voluntarily, while the last type is subject to involuntary contraction. Striated muscles in contrast to smooth muscles (which are subject to involuntary contractions) possess an internal structure of highly organised contractile muscle fibres.

The mimetic muscles are functionally identical to other striated skeletal muscles except the way they arise and insert and hence some structural differences. For instance, a typical skeletal muscle originates from a bone and inserts into a different bone to ensure that upon muscle activation the bones rotate about an axis passing through the joint centre (Fig. 3.5a). In contrast, all mimetic muscle insert in to the skin of the face. The origins of the mimetic muscles, however, could be either from the surface of a bone (e.g. zygomaticus major) (Fig. 3.5b) or another soft tissue such as an aponeurosis (e.g. frontalis) (Fig. 3.5c). Furthermore, the mechanical behaviour of both skeletal and mimetic muscles when subject to internal and external forces is identical.

It must be noted that most engineering structures undergo small deformations. This means the strain, which is a measure of deformation, at any point of the structure can be described as a linear function of the displacement. The latter is the distance between points in the body, before and after deformation, in three dimensions. Furthermore, most engineering materials over small deformations exhibit linear stress-strain characteristics. The stress is a measure of loading and as mentioned strain is a measure of deformation. The stress-strain or simply load-deformation relationship essentially provides the material constitution of the solid body that is being subject to deformation.

The constitutive properties of solid bodies, whether it is biological or engineering, are determined using the data from controlled experiments. An engineering structure that is constructed using linear materials and undergoing small or linear deformations can be mathematically formulated as a linear problem. In contrast, soft tissue structures such as mimetic muscles, in general, undergo large or non-linear deformation. This is primarily because they are relatively compliant. The strain, therefore, becomes a non-linear (quadratic) function of the displacement. Moreover, most biological soft tissues exhibit non-linear constitutive behaviour (stress-strain relationship). For instance, cardiac muscle is a highly non-linear tissue [4] meaning there is exponential increase in stress as strain increases, or in simple terms, the more the body deforms, the higher the force is required to maintain the deformation. Thus, the mathematical problem that arises from soft tissue deformation, in general, is non-linear and at times challenging to solve and often computationally expensive. Figure 3.6 depicts the characteristics of linear and non-linear mechanical deformations.

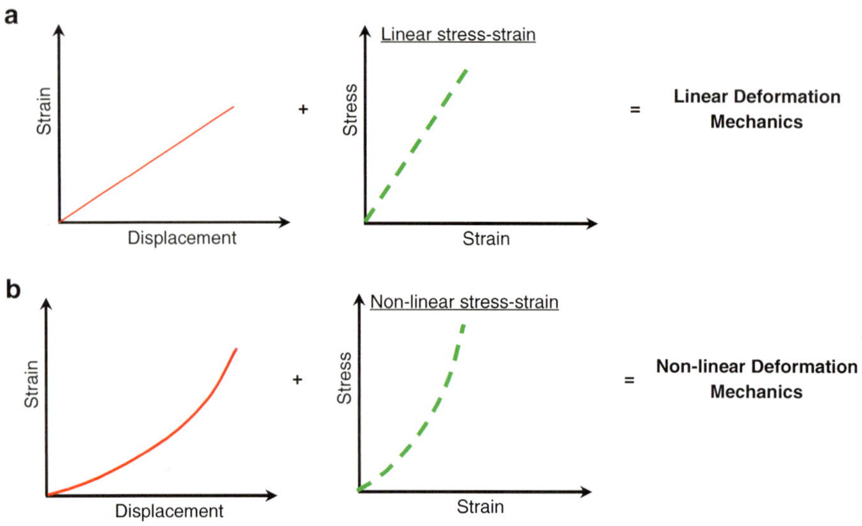

Fig. 3.6 (**a**) Linear strain-displacement deformation and linear stress-strain material. (**b**) Non-linear strain-displacement deformation and non-linear stress-strain material

3.2.2 Structure of Mimetic Muscles

As far as the structure of mimetic muscles is concerned, there are three parameters that need to be taken into account when dealing with their mechanics. Firstly, it is required to have the correct three-dimensional geometry of the undeformed or neutral muscle. Secondly, since the magnitude and direction of internal contractile force that is generated within the muscle is strongly dependent on the fibre arrangement (orientation) in the muscle, it is an important structural parameter. Finally, in order to prescribe the displacement boundary conditions, the knowledge of bony attachment sites is required. The details pertinent these structural parameters of mimetic muscles are discussed next.

Three-Dimensional Geometry of Muscles

All muscles including mimetic muscles found in the human body are true three-dimensional solid structures. Unlike engineering structures, soft tissue counterparts have a complex three-dimensional morphology. In order to determine the deformed shape of these muscles due to muscle activity, it is essential that the initial or undeformed or neutral geometry must be described as accurate as possible. A two-step process is usually adopted to mathematically describe the geometry of a complex structure as anatomically accurate as possible. Firstly, the structure is discretised into smaller and manageable regular-shaped volumes (e.g. tetrahedra or hexahedra in three dimensions). This is one of the fundamental approaches in very popular and widely used numerical discretisation technique called the finite element method [6].

A collection of smaller volumes in computational engineering is called a finite element mesh. The word "mesh" implies an interlaced structure, while "finite element" means simply finite sized elements (volumes). Within a finite element mesh, the elements are connected to each other via nodes. The coordinates (x, y, z) and their (mathematical) derivatives of the nodes serve as the degrees of freedom or the variables that determine the geometry. Secondly, once the mesh nodal degrees of freedoms are available (how they are determined will be discussed shortly), the spatial coordinates (x, y and z) variation within these smaller volumes is then parameterised. This means that the coordinates are described as polynomials of some arbitrary parameters (usually normalised in three dimensions, three such parameters are required) and the mesh nodal degrees of freedom. Figure 3.7 shows the concept of structure geometry discretisation and parameterisation of the discretised geometry.

In order to create discretised geometry of an anatomically complex tissue structure, three-dimensional data are required. These data are usually derived from medical images such as magnetic resonance (MR) images. The process of obtaining discrete data points from images is known as image segmentation in image processing parlance. Certain MR protocols with optimum parameters provide very-high-quality images showing clear muscle boundaries. However, scanning durations for these protocols are prohibitively long. These images can be used with semiautomated or fully automated segmentation techniques to generate data. If the quality of the images is poor, the data is created by manually segmenting the images. The three-dimensional anatomically accurate geometries obtained from medical images such as MR images are patient-specific or individualised as these images represent the anatomy of an individual. There exist other sources to obtain three-dimensional data. Visible human database (https://www.nlm.nih.gov/research/visible/visible_human.html) [7] is one such source of data that contains high-resolution colour tiff (tagged image file format) images. These images have been generated from a 38-year-old male cadaver. There are 1871 images from head to toe at 1 mm intervals in axial plane, and they were made available free of charge in 1994. Since then several published studies involving anatomically based three-dimensional geometries of organs and tissue structures have used the data derived from these images.

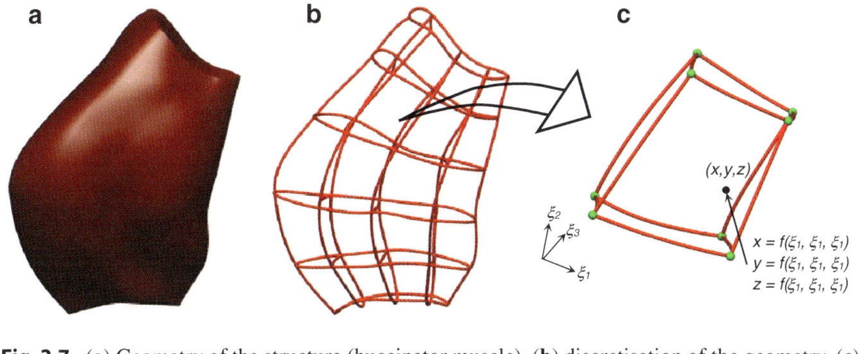

Fig. 3.7 (**a**) Geometry of the structure (buccinator muscle), (**b**) discretisation of the geometry, (**c**) parameterisation of the discretised geometry—ξ_1, ξ_2 and ξ_3 are normalised parameters

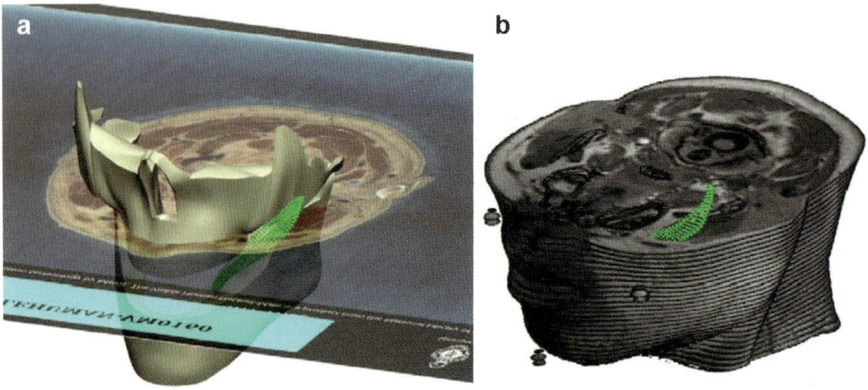

Fig. 3.8 Segmented three-dimensional data of the zygomaticus major muscle from (**a**) visible human images and (**b**) MR images

Note that MR images are in DICOM (digital imaging and communications in medicine) format and images in this format come with a wealth of information (metadata) stored in the header file. These include the spatial location of the image, its orientation, in-plane resolution and host of other useful information. However, other image formats such as tiff or joint photographic experts group (jpeg) do not contain any useful image information that is required for segmentation (three-dimensional data generation). As such this information needs to be supplied with image stack separately; otherwise, the data derived will be meaningless. Figure 3.8 depicts segmented spatial data of skeletal muscle structures from a stack of DICOMs and visible human images.

In order to develop an anatomically accurate three-dimensional geometry of a tissue structure, firstly a subset of the segmented data is used to create a finite element mesh approximating the geometry (Fig. 3.9a). The initial (approximate) finite element mesh is then fitted to all the segmented data (Fig. 3.9b). The fitting process involves determining the mesh nodal degrees of freedom that will best represent the segmented image data. Interested reader is directed to consult references [8, 9] for more details on fitting finite element meshes.

Non-medical images such as visible human photographs generally have a higher resolution (both in-plane as well as in the direction normal to the image plane) and provide better clarity for segmentation. As a result, more data with relatively high accuracy can be generated. The accuracy of the three-dimensional geometry derived from the spatial data is directly proportional to the number of data points. However, it must be noted that not only the number of data points determines overall accuracy of the geometry but the accuracy of segmented data also plays an important role. For instance, a large number of data points with a higher noise (error) will not lead to an accurate three-dimensional geometry. The resolution of medical images (e.g. MR images) on the other hand is relatively poor due to the limitations in the imaging technology itself and logistics involved in imaging a subject.

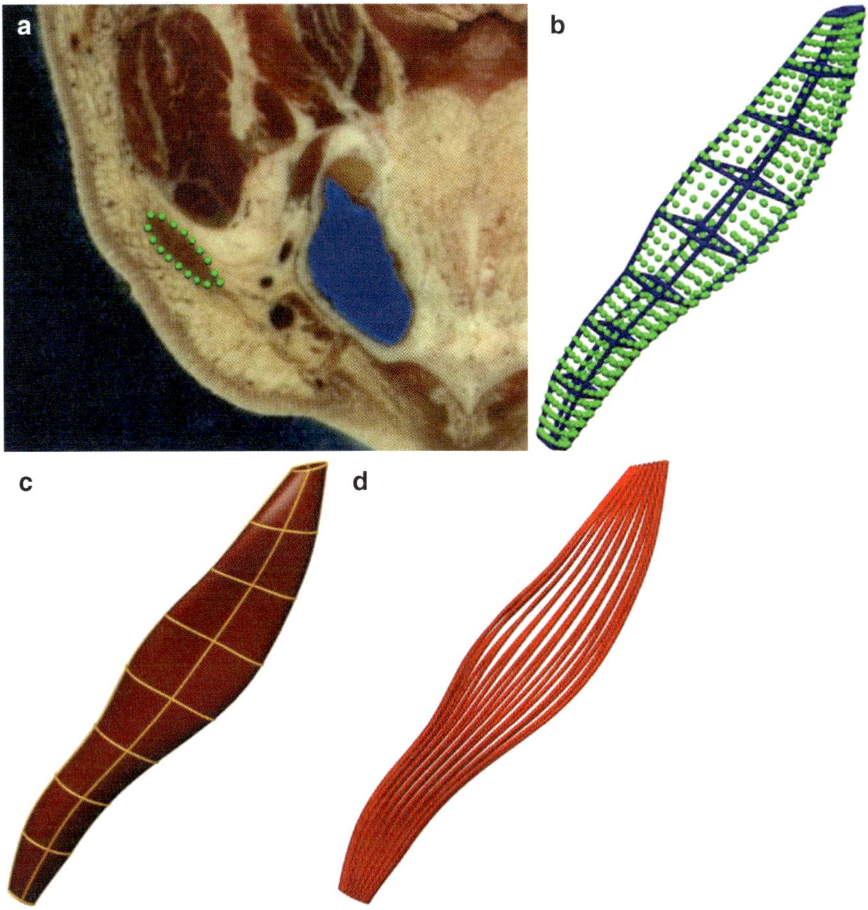

Fig. 3.9 Fitting finite element geometry of zygomaticus major muscle to spatial data derived from visible human images. (**a**) Segmented data from visible human images, (**b**) initial mesh (**c**) fitted mesh, (**d**) fibre/fascicular arrangement (Video 3.1)

Creating several subject-specific and anatomically accurate three-dimensional structures from scratch is cumbersome and time-consuming. Furthermore, fitting needs a large number of data. In order to circumvent this problem, generic geometry can be created from high-quality data (e.g. data from visible human images) and subsequently customised to match subject-specific geometry. In this approach, the number of subject-specific data points required is significantly less than that needed for fitting. There are a number of methods available for customising a generic parameterised geometry [10].

Figure 3.10 depicts the process involved in one such method known as the host mesh customisation method [8, 9]. This is a variant of a technique known as free-form deformation method [11]. Briefly, the generic geometry, which was fitted using

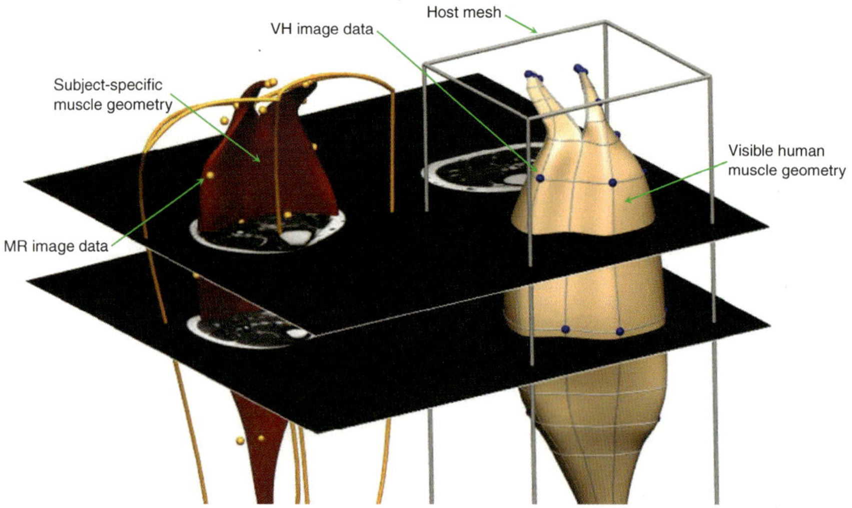

Fig. 3.10 Customisation of the geometry of the gastrocnemius (skeletal muscle) derived from visible human data to create subject-specific geometry using the host mesh method [9] with subject's MR data (Video 3.2)

a large number of smooth (less noisy) data, is embedded in a geometrically simpler mesh known as the host mesh. The next step involves identifying some fiducial points on the generic geometry and corresponding locations (points) on the subject-specific geometry (yet to be created). The latter points are derived from medical images of the subject (e.g. MR images). The host mesh is then morphed to minimise the error between fiducial points. Since the generic geometry is completely embedded in the host mesh (this is one of the requirements in this method), the former deforms with the latter and assumes the shape of the subject-specific structure.

Fibre Organisation in Mimetic Muscles

As mentioned, individual muscle fibres, which usually span over the entire length of the structure, form bundles of fibre known as fascicles. These bundles in turn form the muscle (skeletal or mimetic). The diameter of a myofibre (a multinucleated muscle cell) is in the region of 50–100 mm. Each muscle fibre or muscle cell is sheathed by a connective tissue called endomysium, and each fascicle in a similar manner is surrounded by perimysium. The entire muscle is then surrounded by a connective tissue known as epimysium. Figure 3.11a shows the hierarchical organisation of these constituents within a muscle. Thus, the constitutive properties that describe stress-strain relation are determined by the internal organisation of these constituents (fibres, fascicles and connective tissues) within the muscle.

If the organisation within a muscle fibre or cell is further scrutinised, it contains tightly packed tubular myofibrils that run the entire length of the fibre and are responsible for generating contractile (internal) forces (Fig. 3.11b). The striated appearance of the muscle is due to the alignment of myofibrils within the muscle fibre. The myofibrils can further be divided into repeating functional units called sarcomeres, each of

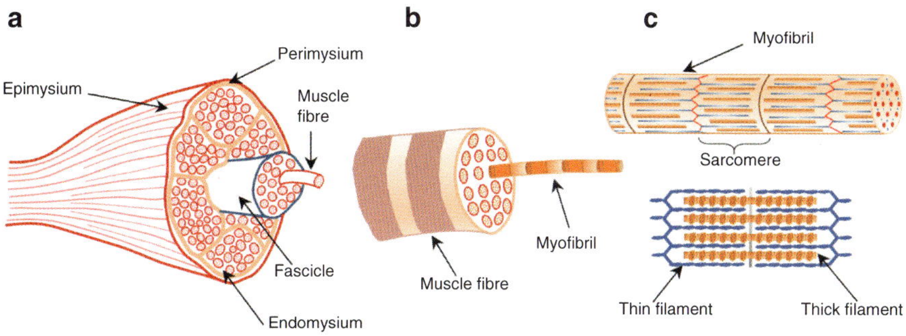

Fig. 3.11 (**a**) Organisation of muscle constituents, (**b**) internal structure of muscle fibres and (**c**) structure of myofibril and sarcomere

which represents a single contractile unit. Each sarcomere contains thick filaments and thin filaments, which are anchored to the Z-disc (Fig. 3.11c). Thin filaments approximately 7 nm in diameter consist primarily of actin, while thick filaments primarily consist of myosin and are approximately about 15 nm in diameter.

The focus is now turned to how the fascicles/fibres are arranged in various mimetic muscles since the direction of the resultant contractile force and ensuing deformed shape of a muscle is a strong function of the fibre/fascicular orientation within it. All muscles that contract voluntarily upon activation by the central nervous system through motor neurons can be categorised into four groups based on the anatomical arrangement of the fibres. **Parallel muscles** are the most abundant type (Fig. 3.12a). These have a common point of attachment, with fascicles running parallel to each other and the force generated aligns with the length direction of the muscle. There are three variants found under this type: flat, fusiform and strap. Usually there is a longer fibre length associated with a fusiform structure, but often the muscle cross section is relatively thin.

Convergent muscles are similar to parallel muscles but relatively broader (Fig. 3.12b). Although the individual fascicles in these muscles do not necessarily run parallel to each other, they have a common point of attachment.

Sphincter muscles are characterised by a circular arrangement of fascicles around an opening (Fig. 3.12c).

In a **pennate or penniform muscle**, the tendon runs through the length of the muscle, with the fascicles attaching obliquely (at an angle) to the tendon (Fig. 3.12d). The fibre or fascicular length is relatively shorter, but penniform muscles have thicker cross-sectional area compared to fusiform counterparts.

These muscles can further be divided as unipennate (single fibre orientation throughout the muscle volume), bipennate (two principal orientations with respect to the line of pull) and multipennate (several orientations within the muscle). Since muscle is a three-dimensional structure, fibre or fascicle angle is defined with respect to its line of action. The latter is the direction of the resultant force of all individual fibre contractile forces.

Most mimetic muscles, with a few exceptions, are parallel muscles. For obvious reasons, there are circular or sphincter muscles around the mouth (orbicularis oris)

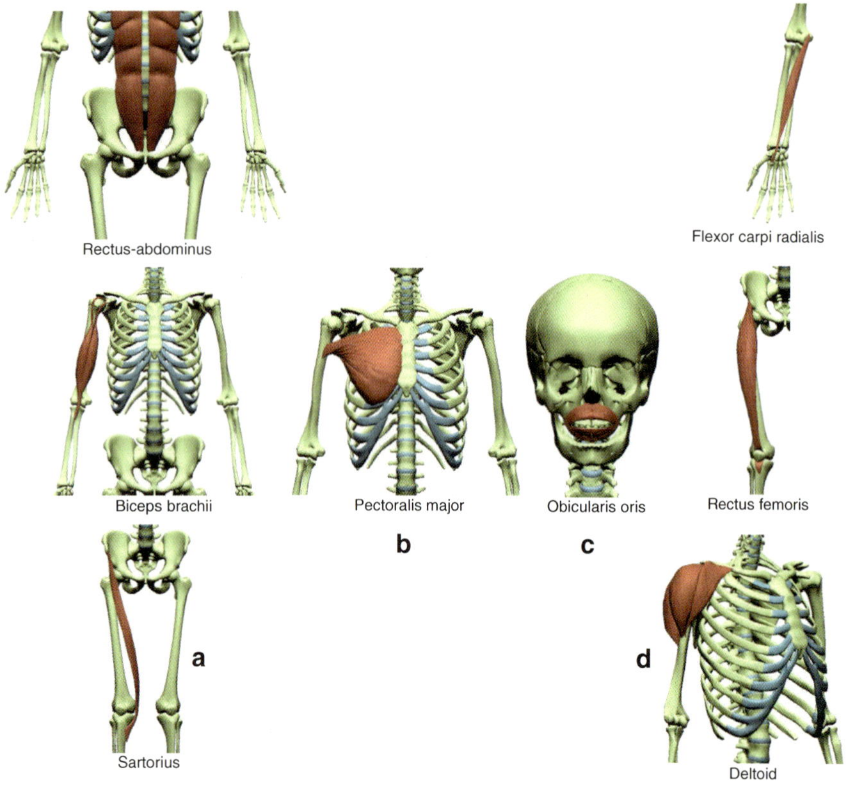

Fig. 3.12 Organisation of muscle fibres. (**a**) **Parallel**: top (flat), middle (fusiform), bottom (strap), (**b**) **convergent**, (**c**) **sphincter** and (**d**) **pennate**—top (unipennate), middle (bipennate), bottom (multipennate)

and eyes (orbicularis oculi). There is a pair of bipennate muscles (buccinators). It not only acts as a mimetic muscle but as a skeletal (masticatory) muscle (causing relative motion between two bony structures) as well. For this reason (dual action), depending on which fibres are activated, the direction and magnitude of the contractile force generated can be controlled. Figure 3.13 shows fibre arrangement and internal force direction in key mimetic muscle volumes.

From the biomechanical point of view, the fibre orientation within the muscle volume is a very important structural parameter. It determines the direction of the contractile force and ensuing facial expressions (facial skin deformations). Figure 3.14 demonstrates how the deformation of the zygomaticus major changes with the fibre angle. The boundary conditions (the origin of the structure) as well as the level of activation (the internal force) in all mechanical simulations shown in Fig. 3.14 were maintained at the same values. Thus, it is clear from the clinical point of view that no procedure should disturb the relative fibre orientations of mimetic muscles.

The foregoing discussion pertinent to fibre arrangement within muscle structures would not be complete if mathematical background behind fibre representation is not explained. It was stated that the geometry of the muscle structure is discretised and parameterised. This enables to represent complex three-dimensional shapes in

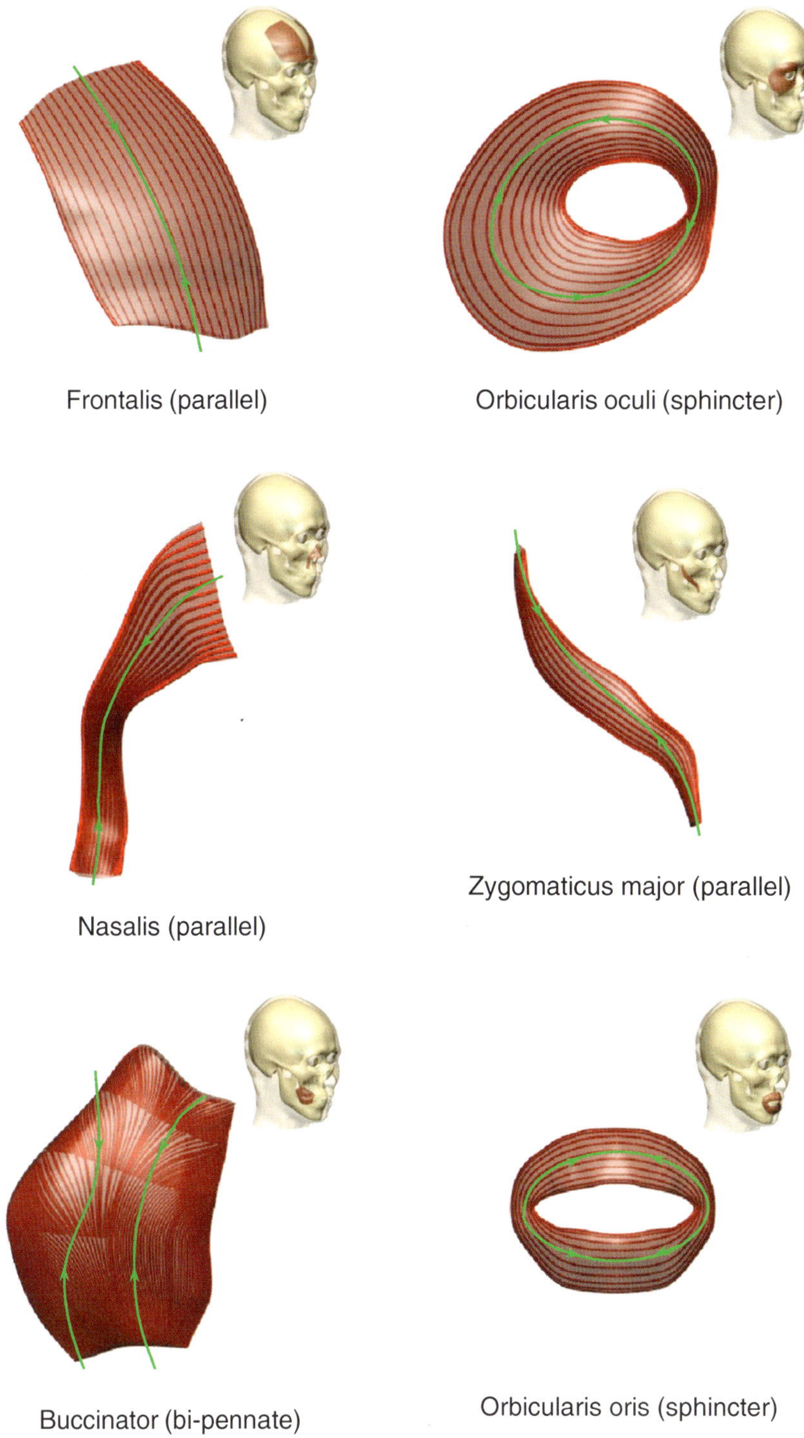

Fig. 3.13 Fibre/fascicular arrangement in mimetic muscles

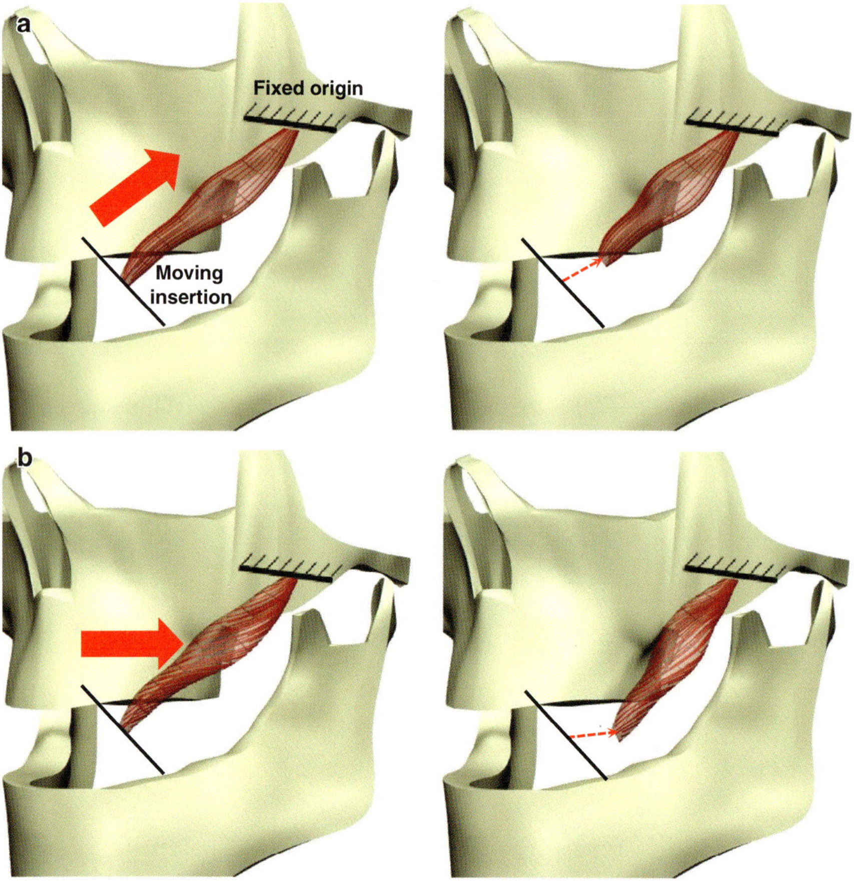

Fig. 3.14 Contraction of zygomaticus major muscle arising from the zygomaticus arch. (**a**) Fibre orientation 0 degrees, (**b**) fibre orientation 20 degrees

a mathematically amenable manner. This means the spatial coordinates at each point of the structure can be generated, and hence the shape of the volume can be constructed (Fig. 3.7). Note that three-dimensional muscle structures are treated as solid continuous media or continua and theoretically, there are an infinite number of points in each continuum. Reverting to the fibre arrangement, the fibre/fascicular orientation or vector direction at each point of the muscle continuum (structure) can also be parameterised in a similar fashion. This is one of the salient features in the finite element method that was mentioned in the preceding section, i.e. any spatially varying quantity (e.g. spatial coordinates, fibre angles, constitutive properties, etc.) can be parameterised after the geometry is discretised.

It was stated at the beginning of Sect. 3.2.2 that there are three key parameters that determine the structure of a mimetic muscle. Although it was not explicitly mentioned that the constitutive properties of the tissue are a structural parameter, they in fact are intimately connected to the structure. As illustrated in Fig. 3.3, constitutive properties of soft tissues, especially muscles, depend on the way the fibres are organised within the tissue.

Attachments of Mimetic Muscles

Another important structural parameter in mimetic or facial muscle deformation is its attachments, in particular, the origin. It has already been mentioned that the primary difference between a skeletal and mimetic muscle is the way they attach (Fig. 3.5). The latter type of muscles arises from a bone or another soft tissue structure but always inserts into the skin. When a muscle originates from a bone, the attachment site prescribes the displacement boundary conditions during mechanical deformation.

Figure 3.15a shows the contraction of the zygomaticus major, a mimetic muscle, with one end (origin) fixed and the other end free to move. A contraction of a skeletal muscle (biceps brachii) is shown in Fig. 3.15b with both ends fixed (isometric contraction). Note that there is always a movement around the insertion area when a mimetic muscle is activated while it is not uncommon to have stationary conditions at the both end of a skeletal muscle during activation (contraction). For instance, when a weight is held in hand, the internal muscle forces are generated to sustain the equilibrium, but there is no relative or absolute movement of the attachment sites in space.

3.2.3 Function of Mimetic Muscles

Having discussed the structural parameters of mimetic muscles and their implications on mechanics, the focus is now turned to their functional aspects. In particular, it is important to understand how the contractile force is generated within the muscle and how it can be quantified using the level of activation instigated by the central nervous system and its relation to other structural parameters such as fibre length.

Although skeletal muscles have multiple functions, mimetic muscles are primarily responsible for generating facial expressions. The superficial fascia enveloping the mimetic muscle has intimate connections with the skin. As a result contractions of mimetic muscles due to internal force generation lead to prominent surface deformations that form different facial expressions. For instance, the forces in zygomaticus muscles draw the mouth corners laterally and superiorly during smiling while the levator muscles elevate the lips. The depressor muscles in the mandibular region draw the lips downwards upon activation to show the teeth, and the mentalis contracts to purse the lower lip.

It was already mentioned in the preceding section that muscle fibres or muscle cells contain myofibrils which are made of repeating functional units called sarcomeres. Each sarcomere in turn contains thick and thin protein filaments called actin and myosin, respectively (Fig. 3.11c). When muscle cells contract, these overlapping filaments do not change their size; instead, they slide pass each other and generate a tensile force within the muscle. This is known as the sliding filament mechanism. The theory pertaining to sliding filaments was first introduced by

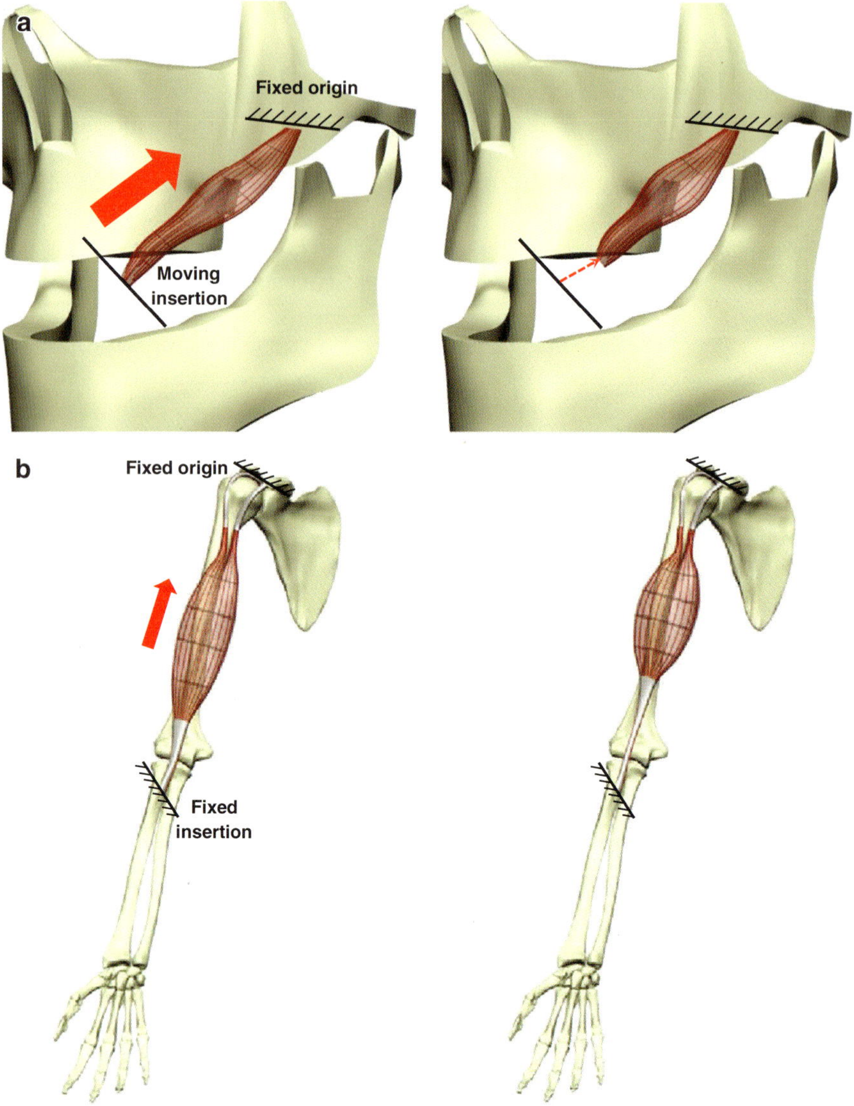

Fig. 3.15 Contraction of muscles subject to different boundary conditions (attachments). (**a**) Mimetic muscle (zygomaticus major) with fixed origin, (**b**) skeletal muscle (biceps brachii) with both origin and insertion fixed

Andrew Huxley and Rolf Niedergerke in 1954. Mimetic muscle contractions are neurogenic (activated by a nerve signal originated from the brain) as they require input from motor neurons to produce muscle contractions. In contrast, the involuntary contractions occurring in smooth and cardiac muscles are myogenic meaning the contractions are initiated by muscle cells themselves. A single motor neuron is able to innervate multiple muscle fibres causing them to contract at the same time.

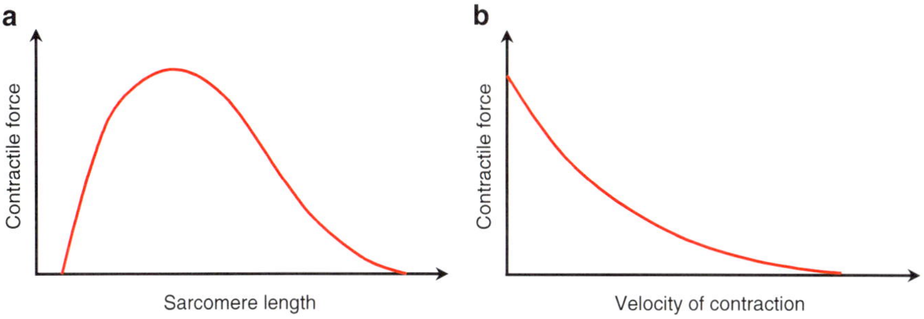

Fig. 3.16 Contractile force against (**a**) sarcomere length and (**b**) contractile velocity

Since all facial (mimetic) muscles undergo active voluntary contractions, the direction of the internal contractile or tensile force which determines how the muscle deforms is dictated by the fibre/fascicle orientation within the muscle volume. The magnitude of the contractile force generated by sliding filaments in myofibrils is dependent on the degree of filament overlap (i.e. sarcomere/fibre/muscle length) and how fast the sarcomere/fibre/muscle length changes. Furthermore, the higher the level of activation at a given fibre length, the larger the generated force will be. Mathematically this force can be described by a Hill-type model which is a phenomenological model formulated based on experimental observations.

At sarcomere level (Fig. 3.11c), the relationship between the contractile force generated and sarcomere length typically shows a quadratic variation (Fig. 3.15a). Since mechanical analyses on striated muscles are predominantly static or quasi-static, the dependence of the contractile force on velocity is usually not considered in three-dimensional continuum mechanics. However, the contractile force is inversely proportional to the velocity of contractions of sarcomere (Fig. 3.16b) [12].

Another variable that needs to be considered for determining the contractile force generated within the muscle is the degree of activation. The force-length and force-velocity functional parameters discussed above did not consider the degree of activation. Based on the required muscle force for a given task, the central nervous system determines how many fibres of the muscle need to be stimulated. This process is called motor unit recruitment. A motor unit has one motor neuron that sends signals to several fibre strands that it innervates. A muscle contains several such motor units. The activation of one motor neuron results in a weak but distributed muscle contractile force. The activation of more motor neurons results in more muscle fibres being activated and therefore a stronger muscle contraction. The higher the recruitment, the stronger the muscle contractile force will be.

3.3 Mathematical Representation of the Three-Dimensional Facial Anatomy

In the preceding section, biomechanics of individual mimetic muscles was discussed with regard to its structure and function. The initial undeformed or neutral anatomically based geometry, fascicular arrangement within the muscle body, its constitutive properties and attachments determine the mechanical structure. As far as the function of a muscle is concerned, the contractile force is the key parameter which in turn is responsible for facial expressions. As was mentioned earlier, facial movements are generated by coordinated actions of over 40 muscles in the face. Therefore, the next logical step is to look at the structure and function of the face as a whole.

Figure 3.17 shows the three-dimensional anatomically based whole face geometry derived from two different sources of data. The finite element (discretised and parameterised) geometry in Fig. 3.17 was constructed using the visible human [6] segmented data, while Fig. 3.18 depicts a finite element geometry constructed using the data from MR images of a healthy 25-year-old male volunteer.

It was stated in Sect. 3.1 (Fig. 3.9) that subject-specific facial geometry can be created from generic geometries such as the one derived from the visible human data [7]. Figure 3.19 shows a finite element facial geometry of a healthy 28-year-old male volunteer created using the host mesh-based free-form deformation method [8] starting with the visible human face as the generic geometry. The data for the customisation have been derived from visible human images and volunteer's MR images [1]. In Fig. 3.20, creation of a three-dimensional facial geometry of a female volunteer is illustrated using the same technique. Here the male volunteer's geometry serves as the generic or original geometry. The MR image data of the male volunteer and structured light data of the female volunteer from the Bosphorus 3D Face Database [13] have been used for the customisation.

Figure 3.21 shows the fibre/fascicular arrangement in facial muscles corresponding to the geometries in Figs. 3.17 and 3.18.

It is theoretically possible to determine the mechanical action of individual muscles and then infer the ensuing deformation (expression) of the entire face. However, this approach results in a complex and computationally expensive mathematical problem. One of the reasons for this difficulty is to handle contact interaction between muscles. It has been reported in an underwater ultrasonographic study [14] that upon activation, adjacent mimetic muscles act in unison rather than individually and do not show any relative motion between them.

Furthermore, it is a well-established fact that most superficial mimetic muscles are connected to the superficial musculo-aponeurotic system or SMAS. Thus, in order to make the problem at hand computationally manageable, a single three-dimensional continuum incorporating all structural and functional properties of individual mimetic muscles and other soft tissues can be utilised. This single continuous tissue structure will therefore contain the geometry, fibre/fascicular orientation, constitutive properties and attachment sites each soft tissue structures enveloped by it. Interested reader is referred to the work by Wu et al. [15] for the details (e.g. mathematical formulation, etc.) of this approach.

Facial retaining ligaments and muscles attachment points/sites need to be correctly included in the single continuum geometry to ensure the deformation due to muscle activation is physiologically correct. In other words, bone-muscle attachment sites prescribe the displacement or Dirichlet boundary conditions for the problem at hand. Spatial locations of the tissue geometry where displacement boundary

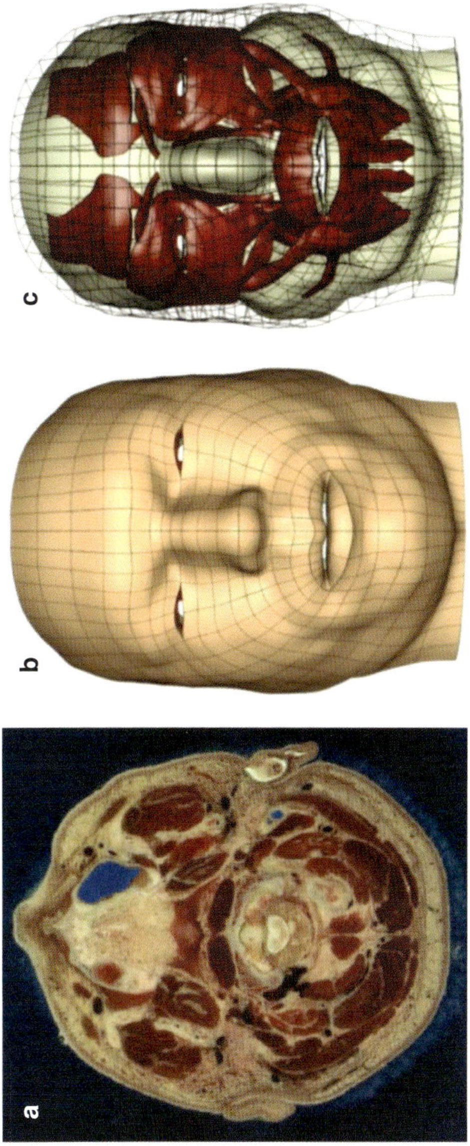

Fig. 3.17 Anatomically based three-dimensional finite element mesh of the face derived from visible human image data. (**a**) Visible human image (cryosection), (**b**) finite element mesh of the face, (**c**) three-dimensional internal tissue structures

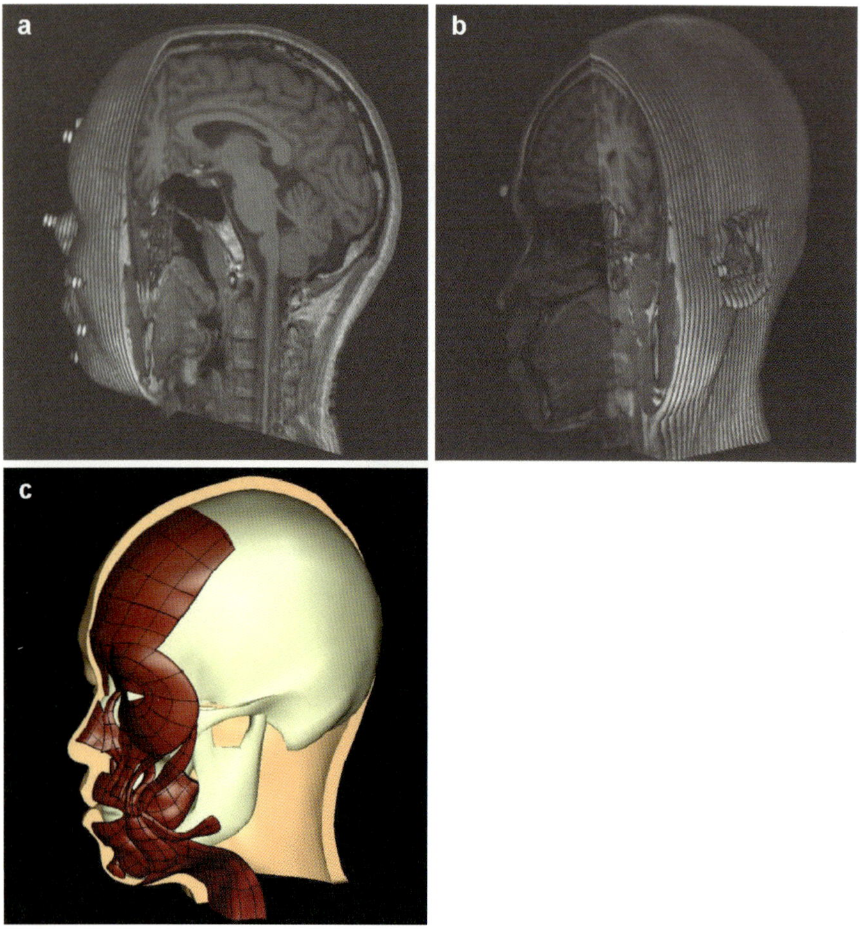

Fig. 3.18 Anatomically based three-dimensional finite element mesh of the face derived from the MR image data of a male volunteer. (**a**, **b**) Cutaway views of MR image stack, (**c**) three-dimensional mesh

conditions are required to be applied are depicted in Fig. 3.22. Shown in Fig. 3.23 is a retaining ligament whose three-dimensional geometry was derived from a 56-year-old male volunteer's MR image data acquired in the supine position.

Beneath the superficial soft tissue layer that predominantly contains mimetic muscles and retaining ligaments, there exists a deep tissue layer. The later layer consists of masticatory muscles, salivary glands and fat pads. If the superficial layer is treated as a single continuous tissue, then it is necessary to impose suitable constraints to ensure that there is no interpenetration between the superficial and deep layers. Furthermore, to prevent interpenetration between lower and upper lips as well as lower and upper eyelids, constraint must be imposed. As far as the superficial and deep layers contact interaction is concerned, certain areas of the former must be allowed to slide over the latter. Therefore, this type of interaction between two solid bodies is called sliding

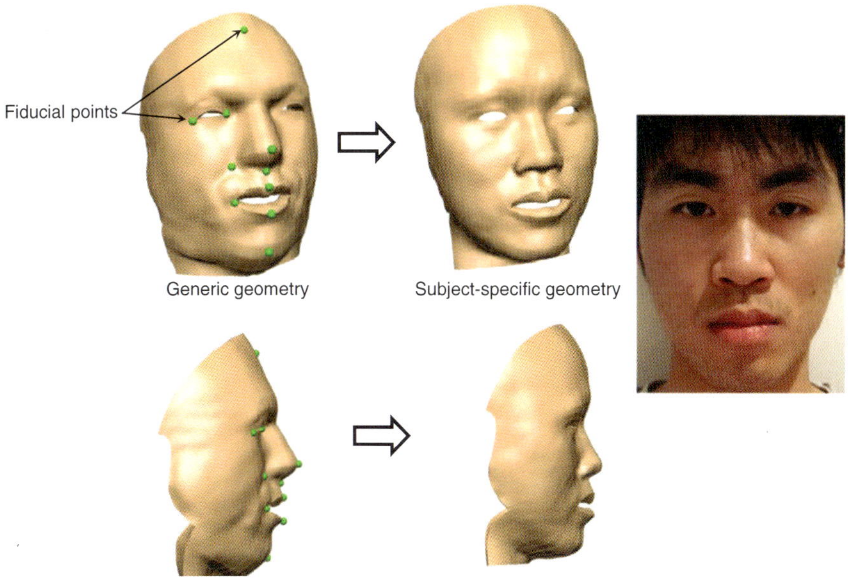

Fig. 3.19 Three-dimensional facial geometry of a male volunteer created from the facial geometry of visible human using the host mesh technique with visible human image data and volunteer's MR image data (*Adapted from Hung et al.* [1])

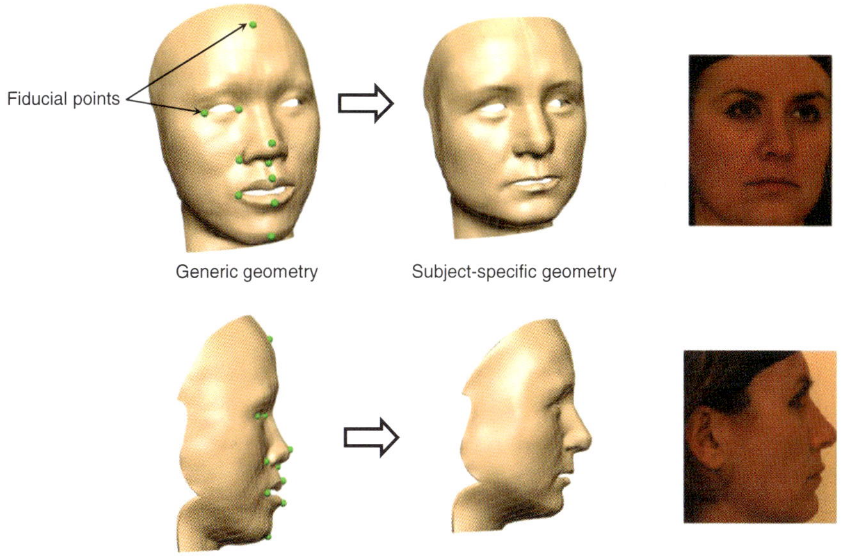

Fig. 3.20 Three-dimensional facial geometry of a female volunteer created from the facial geometry of a male volunteer using the host mesh technique with male volunteer's MR image data and female volunteer's structured light facial data (*Adapted from Hung et al.* [1])

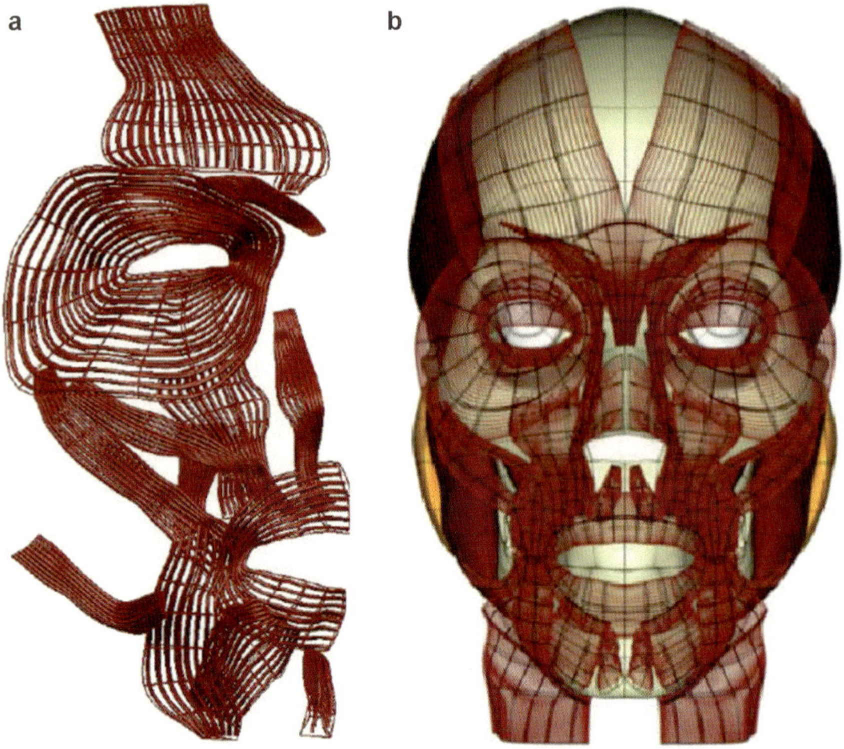

Fig. 3.21 Fibre arrangement in anatomically based three-dimensional geometry of the face derived from (**a**) visible human image data and (**b**) MR image data of a male volunteer

contact (i.e. sliding one body over the other and no interpenetration between them). Note that some regions of the deep layer have bony non-deformable structures (mandible and maxilla) and the rest is deformable tissue. Figure 3.24a shows the locations where contact constraints need to be imposed to prevent interpenetration between the upper and lower lips and the upper and lower eyelids. The contact between the superficial and deep tissue layers is shown in Fig. 3.24b.

Finally, the discussion pertaining to the biomechanics of the whole face is closed by explaining how the constitutive properties of various tissue types are handled. Since the human face is a structurally complex unit, it contains several soft tissue types with distinct constitutive properties. Based on their constitutive properties, three main groups of soft tissue structures can be identified. They are the skin, subcutaneous fat and muscles. From a mechanical strength point of view, the skin that consists of several sub-layers is the stiffest, while the subcutaneous fat offers the least resistance to deformation [18]. Again, if the superficial layer is represented by a single tissue layer (continuum) with all mimetic muscles, subcutaneous fat and skin embedded in it, then heterogeneity as well as directional dependence must be described as accurate as possible. Note that material property heterogeneity and their directional dependence are two different aspects. For instance, properties of two muscle regions embedded in the superficial layer can have identical directional

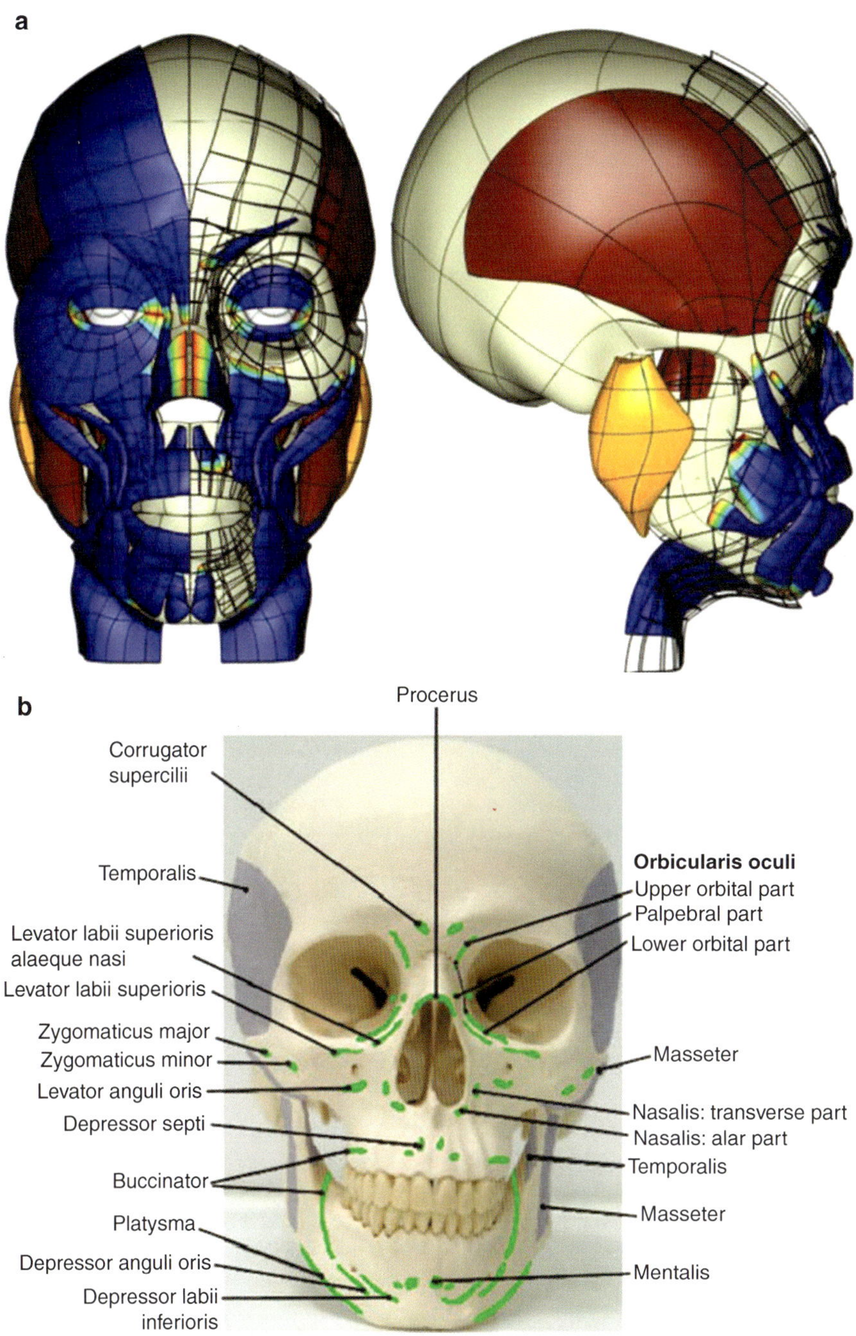

Fig. 3.22 Displacement boundary conditions for tissue continuum. (**a**) Muscle attachment points/sites indicated in red (*Adapted from Wu et al.* [16]). (**b**) Muscle attachment areas to the facial skeleton (*Adapted from Prendagast* [17])

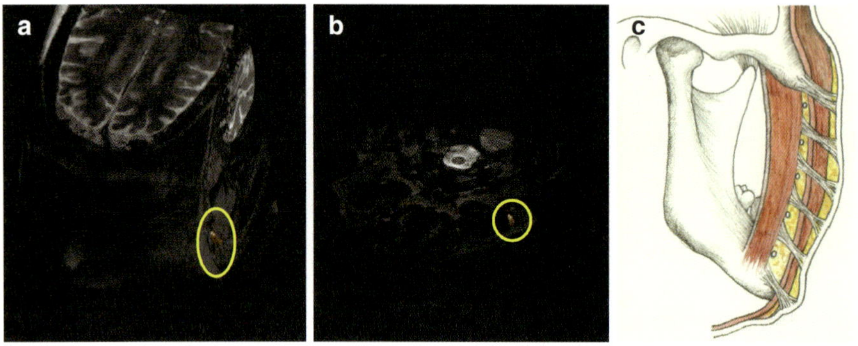

Fig. 3.23 Retaining ligaments. (**a**) Sagittal plane view. (**b**) Transverse plane view. (**c**) A schematic view

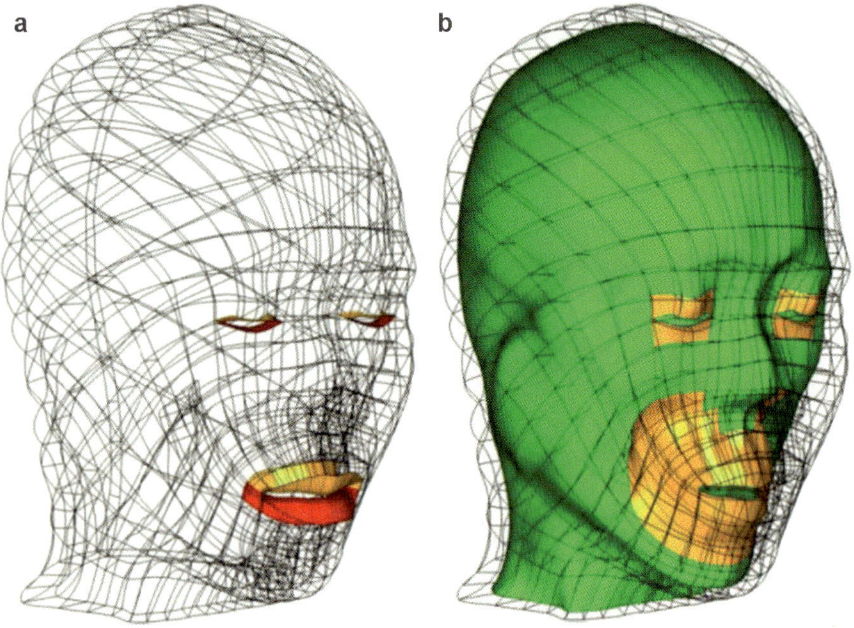

Fig. 3.24 Contact constraints. (**a**) Lips and eyelids. (**b**) Superficial and deep layers—green (sliding and no interpenetration), gold (no interpenetration only) (*Adapted from Wu et al.* [16])

dependence (e.g. along the fibre direction), but the coefficients associated with the directions could be different. Nonetheless, once the geometry of the tissue layer was discretised and parameterised (see Sect. 3.2.2.1), material heterogeneity and direction dependence can be efficiently handled by treating these as spatially varying field variables (see Sect. 3.2.2.2). How constitutive property heterogeneity within the facial superficial layer is mathematically handled is described in the work by Mithraratne et al. [19].

3.4 Facial Expression Simulations

Anatomically, accurate facial geometry (discretised and parameterised) with all biomechanical characteristics (fibre orientation, appropriate constitutive properties, boundary conditions and constraints) incorporated in it that deforms upon muscle activation (loading) satisfying the governing laws (physics) is called a biomechanical computational model. Such a computational model can be an effective tool to gain more insight into how facial tissue structures functionally interact. However, the computational model's ability to predict the mechanics of the three-dimensional face must be tested. This is called model validation and is performed against experimental data usually acquired under controlled conditions. Validating anatomically based three-dimensional biomechanical computational model of the face against measured (structured light) data for four expressions (smile (mouth closed), smile (mouth opened), sad, terror) is described in the work by Wu et al. [16, 20]. Figure 3.25 shows the measured expressions and their biomechanical model predictions of the four expressions.

Once the computational model is validated against experimental data, as stated earlier, it can be used to investigate various what-if scenarios. The three-dimensional biomechanical finite element computational model developed by Chabanas and Payan [21] demonstrates how their model can be integrated into a surgical simulator for plastic and maxillofacial surgeries. Their aim was to predict the patient's facial

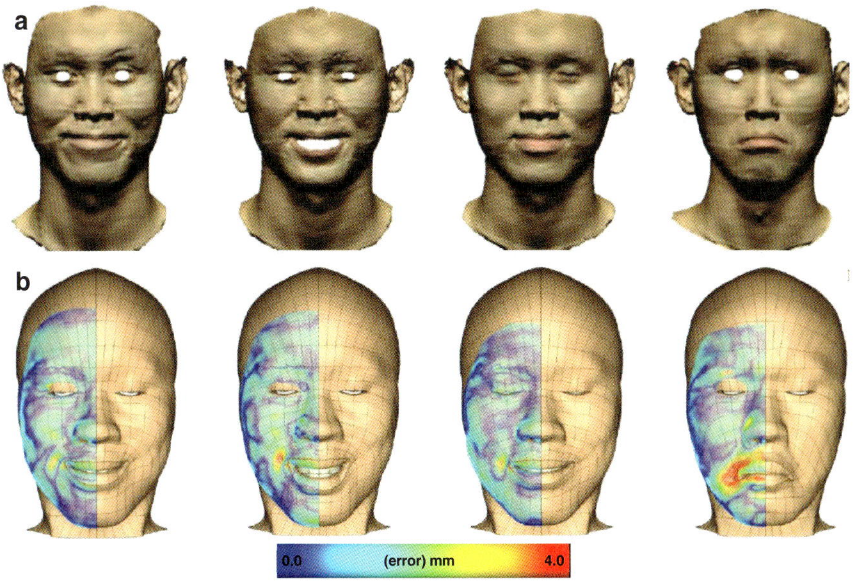

Fig. 3.25 Comparison of predicted deformation (expressions) against measured data. (**a**) Three-dimensional surface data acquired using a structured light scanner. (**b**) Predicted expressions from the biomechanical model with the error between predicted and measured deformation superimposed (*Adapted from Wu et al.* [16])

deformations following the repositioning of the mandible and maxilla. The model was developed to provide the surgeon with a tool to plan maxillary and mandibular osteotomies using a three-dimensional patient-specific geometry constructed from computed tomography (CT) images and capable of predicting: (a) facial aesthetics due to passive deformation of soft tissues after bone repositioning and (b) active deformations of the face under muscle actions.

Equally, a three-dimensional biomechanical model which deals with mimetic muscle deformations discussed in this chapter can be employed to simulate and review vector and contour congruent facelift procedures described in Chap. 4. For instance, the effect of repositioning mimetic muscle insertions on static (neutral) and dynamic (deformed) face can be investigated. The term "vector" implies the direction of tissue deformation, while "contour" defines the shape of the facial soft tissue composite. It is important to remember that both terms are used in three-dimensional context. As described earlier these two variables (the direction and degree of tissue deformation) following a facelift are determined by the structure and function of soft tissues in the face.

Figures 3.26 and 3.27 show predicted facial expressions (deformations) due to active contractions of various mimetic muscles reported by Wu et al. [16] and Chabanas and Payan [21], respectively. Muscle activation levels used to simulate the facial expressions depicted in Fig. 3.26 are summarised in Table 3.1.

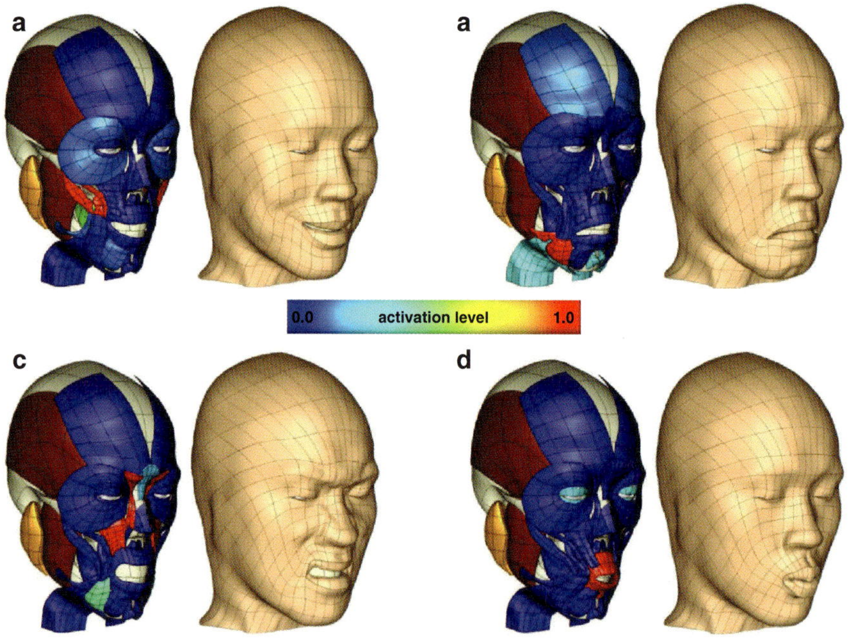

Fig. 3.26 Facial expressions predicted using a computational biomechanical model of the human face with active contraction of mimetic muscles. Colour (blue, 0; red, 1) of the mimetic muscles indicates the level of muscle activation. (**a**) Joy (smile), (**b**) sadness, (**c**) snarl, (**d**) kissing (*Adapted from Wu et al.* [16])

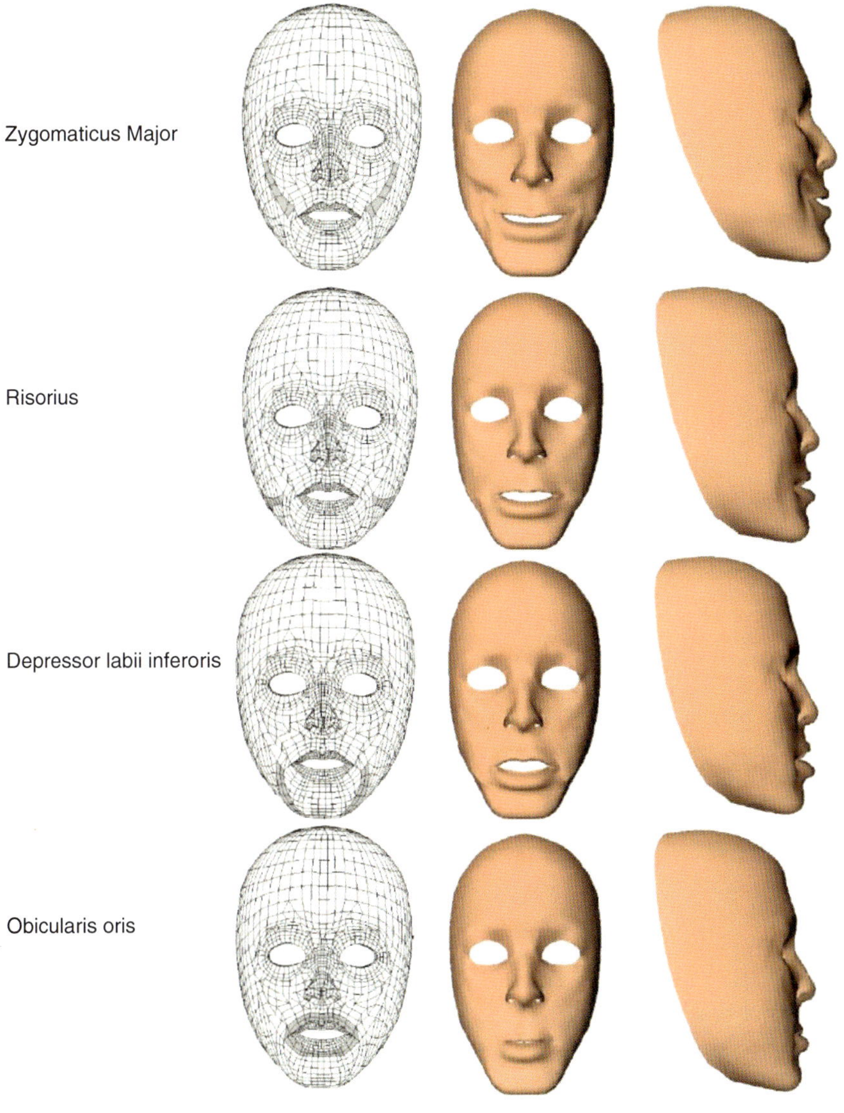

Fig. 3.27 Facial expressions predicted using a computational biomechanical model of the human face with active contraction of mimetic muscles (*Adapted from Chabanas and Payan* [21])

Although the validated biomechanical computational model is a useful tool from the clinical point of view, one of its major drawbacks is its computational cost and hence the time taken to solve the model equations, especially if the tissues undergo non-linear deformations. That is the case for most of the time as mimetic muscles are relatively compliant and exhibit non-linear stress-strain properties. Moreover, the interaction due to contact between tissues (e.g. superficial and deep layers of the

Table 3.1 Muscle activation levels for the expression shown in Fig. 3.26

Expression	Active muscle and the level of activation (in brackets)
Joy	Buccinator ($\alpha = 0.5$), depressor labii inferioris ($\alpha = 0.1$), levator anguli oris ($\alpha = 1.0$), orbital orbicularis oculi ($\alpha = 0.1$), risorius ($\alpha = 0.1$), zygomaticus major ($\alpha = 1.0$) and zygomaticus minor ($\alpha = 1.0$)
Sadness	Corrugator supercilii ($\alpha = 1.0$), depressor anguli oris ($\alpha = 1.0$), frontalis ($\alpha = 0.1$), mentalis ($\alpha = 0.3$) and risorius ($\alpha = 1.0$)
Snarl	Corrugator ($\alpha = 1.0$), depressor anguli oris ($\alpha = 0.4$), depressor supercilii ($\alpha = 1.0$), levator labii superioris ($\alpha = 1.0$), levator labii superioris alaeque nasi ($\alpha = 1.0$) and procerus ($\alpha = 0.2$)
Kissing	Palpebral orbicularis oculi ($\alpha = 0.3$) and orbicularis oris ($\alpha = 1.0$)

face) is, in general, non-linear, and hence several highly non-linear equations need to be solved. A typical prediction of such model with a high-end desktop computer can take more than 2 h per simulation. Thus, if the model is to be used for predicting several what-if scenarios to plan a certain procedure, it can easily take hundreds of hours. Furthermore, analysis of the results from a large number of simulations is a time-consuming cumbersome task.

Validated computational models, however, can be used to generate numerical data (simulation results). This is akin to conducting an experiment in a laboratory and acquiring experimental data. In theory, a model can be used to generate numerical data for infinite number of scenarios. The numerical data that are obtained from a computational model can be divided into two groups: the inputs and outputs. For instance, the inputs are the degrees of freedom or spatial coordinates of the undeformed three-dimensional geometry (discretised and parameterised) of the face, activation levels of each muscle, etc. The outputs are spatial coordinates of the deformed face. So, using a computational model, it is possible to generate hundreds of thousands of input-output (numerical) data. With these data, it is possible to formulate a multi-input/multi-output statistical model. This type of mathematical model is known as a meta-model, which is a simplified model of the original computationally expensive mathematical model. The original model (e.g. non-linear biomechanical model of the face) is a physics-based computational model, which consists of non-linear differential and algebraic equations. The meta-model, on the other hand, is an algebraic model, and its parameters are obtained by solving a linear system of equations. Once the parameters are identified, the deformed state can be very quickly obtained (usually in seconds) for a given input/s (e.g. muscle activation level).

There are a number of methods available to construct a multivariate meta-model from numerical or experimental data. Each method has its own merits and flaws depending on the nature of the data. Wu et al. [22] developed a partial least squares regression (PLSR) meta-model to reproduce the facial expressions obtained from a detailed physics-based biomechanical model [19]. Figure 3.28 shows the results from both models and the error in the deformation predicted by the meta-model with respect to the biomechanical model.

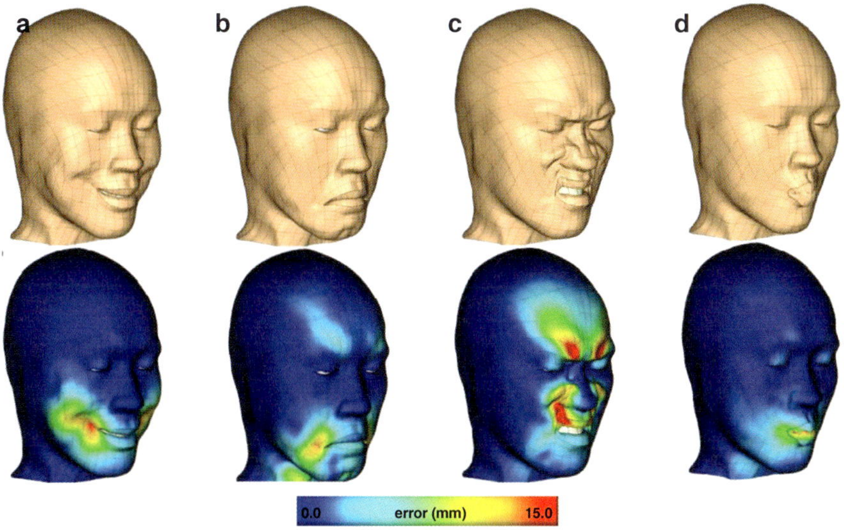

Fig. 3.28 Comparison of facial expressions predicted using a physics-based (biomechanical) computational model and meta-model of the human face with active contraction of mimetic muscles. Error is calculated with respect to the former model. (**a**) Joy (smile), (**b**) sadness, (**c**) snarl, (**d**) kissing (*Adapted from Wu et al.* [22])

3.5 Concluding Remarks

In this chapter, biomechanics of mimetic muscles and the whole face was discussed in detail. In particular, mathematical formulation of structural and functional aspects of these units from mechanical point of view was examined. The structural and functional properties of the facial soft tissue composite play an important role in vector and contour congruent facelift procedures described in this book (Chap. 4) as they determine the static (at rest) and dynamic (smiling, fright, terror, etc.) shape of the face following a procedure. Traditionally these procedures had been viewed from a two-dimensional perspective. The two-dimensional view of the three-dimensional face naturally tends to ignore its volume and treat the face as a flattened object. This can often lead to a non-congruent facelift. Since most mimetic muscles insert at the "changeover junctions" or "pilasters" (Chap. 2), non-congruent procedures distort the three-dimensional shape of the face. Vector and contour congruent facelifts, on the other hand, restore the mimetic muscle insertions and latitudes correctly in three dimensions to give a firm, full and youthful appearance of the face (Chap. 2). In order to perform a congruent facelift, the surgeon must be well conversant with the three-dimensional anatomy. However, visualising a structurally and functionally complex unit such as the three-dimensional face and making correct surgical decisions to ensure vector and contour congruent outcome are difficult tasks. To that end, an anatomically based and subject-specific biomechanical computational model of the face or its meta-model counterpart is a valuable clinical tool that can be used by the surgeon to make an informed decision. Since meta-models are significantly faster than physics-based biomechanical models and relatively easy to run on a standard desktop machine, the former will be the natural choice for clinical applications. However, it must be remembered that a validated biomechanical model is still required to generate numerical data for the meta-model.

References

1. Hung APL, Wu T, Hunter P, Mithraratne K (2015) A framework for generating anatomically detailed subject-specific human facial models for biomechanical simulations. Vis Comput 31(5):527–539
2. Schuenke M, Schulte E, Schumacher U, Ross L, Lamperti E, Voll M (2010) Head and neuroanatomy. Thieme Medical Publishers, New York, NY
3. Aston J, Steinbrech D, Walden J (2009) Aesthetic plastic surgery. Elsevier Health Sciences, Amsterdam
4. Hunter PJ (1995) Myocardial constitutive laws for continuum mechanics models of the heart. In: Sideman S, Beyer R (eds) Molecular and subcellular cardiology. Plenum Press, New York, NY, pp 303–318
5. Abbott BC, Baskin RJ (1962) Volume changes in frog muscle during contraction. J Physiol 161:379–391
6. Reddy JN (2005) An introduction to the finite element method, 3rd edn. McGraw Hill, New York, NY
7. Ackerman MJ (1998) The visible human project. Proc IEEE 86:504–511
8. Bradley CP, Pullan AJ, Hunter PJ (1997) Geometric modelling of the human torso using cubic hermite elements. Ann Biomed Eng 25:96–111
9. Fernandez JW, Tawhai MH, Mithraratne P, Thrupp SF, Hunter PJ (2004) Anatomically based geometric modelling of the musculo-skeletal system and other organs. Biomech Model Mechanobiol 2:139–155
10. Mithraratne K, Hunter PJ (2006) Customisation of anatomically based musculoskeletal structures. In: Proceedings of the ICMMB-15, Singapore, 6–8 December 2006, pp 467–470
11. Sederberg TW, Parry SR (1986) Free-form deformation of solid geometric models. ACM Comput Graph 20(4):151–160
12. Morgan DL, Claflin DR, Julian FJ (1991) Tension as a function of sarcomere length and velocity of shortening in single skeletal muscle fibres of the frog. J Physiol 441:719–732
13. Savran A, Alyüz N, Dibekliöglu H, Çeliktutan O, Gökberk B, Akarun L (2008) Bosphorus database for 3D face analysis. In: The First COST 2101 Workshop on Biometrics and Identity Management (BIOID 2008). Roskilde University, Denmark, pp 7–9
14. Wu T, Mithraratne K, Sagar M, Hunter PJ (2010) Characterizing facial tissue sliding using ultrasonography. In: Lim CT, Goh JCH (eds) 6th World Congress of Biomechanics, IFMBE Proceedings, vol 31, pp 1566–1569
15. Wu T, Hung AP-L, Hunter PJ, Mithraratne K (2013) Modelling facial expressions: a framework for simulating nonlinear soft tissue deformations using embedded 3D muscles. Finite Elem Anal Design 76:63–70
16. Wu T, Hung A, Mithraratne K (2014) Generating facial expressions using an anatomically accurate biomechanical Model. IEEE Trans Vis Comput Graph 20(11):1519–1529
17. Prendagast PM (2012) Anatomy of the face and neck. In: Shiffman MA, Di Giuseppe A (eds) Cosmetic surgery – art and techniques. Springer, Berlin, pp 29–45
18. Hung A, Mithraratne K, Sagar M (2009) Multilayer soft tissue continuum model: towards realistic simulation of facial expressions. World Acad Sci Eng Tech 54:134–138

19. Mithraratne K, Hung A, Sagar M, Hunter PJ (2010) An efficient heterogeneous continuum model to simulate active contraction of facial soft tissue structures. IFMBE Proc 31:1024–1027
20. Wu T, Hunter PJ, Mithraratne K (2013) Simulating and validating facial expressions using an anatomically accurate biomechanical model derived from MRI data: towards fast and realistic generation of animated characters, GRAPP 2013. In: Proceedings of the International Conference on Computer Graphics Theory and Applications and International Conference on Information Visualization Theory and Applications, Barcelona, Spain, pp 267–272
21. Chabanas M, Payan Y (2000) A 3D finite element model of the human face for simulation in plastic and maxilla-facial surgery. In: Delp SL, DiGioia AM, Jaramaz B (eds) MICCAI 2000. Springer, Berlin, pp 1068–1075
22. Wu T, Martens H, Hunter P, Mithraratne K (2014) Emulating facial biomechanics using multivariate partial least squares surrogate models. Int J Num Methods Biomed Eng 30(11): 1103–1120

4 Operative Procedures

4.1 Introduction

The aged face is graced by sagging skin and soft tissue characterised by a lax neck with bilateral vertical folds in front. The ageing stigmas consist of progressive upper cheek ptosis, lower eyelid-cheek sulcus, nasolabial folds, marionette deformity, jowls, anterior platysma bands and obtuse cervical-mental angle as seen in Fig. 4.1a–c.

These ageing stigmas are predetermined by the support system of fibrous ligament/septa developed for the mid- and lower face which consists of two horizontal rows of ligaments/septa at the top and bottom of the mid-/lower face complex, buttressed by an oblique row of ligament/septa (masseteric ligament and septa) at the front/side plane changeover junction (Fig. 4.2a, b).

In the young, this tight ligament/septa system runs through the full dense intervening soft tissue to be inserted into the deep dermal surface after penetrating the SMAS. This soft tissue and packing fat are enclosed by tight tense well-circumscribed compartments in the young (Figs. 4.3a, b and 4.4).

This tight compartment system has some weak points as is demonstrated in Figs. 4.3a and 4.4. These deficiencies generate the predictable stigma pattern of the old face. The mandibular septa, platysma-auricular ligament and intervening dense adhesions are an effective bulwark against the downward descent of the compartment above. In our clinical operative experience, we do not find evidence of herniation of the lateral temporal cheek fat compartment extending below the mandibular border [1]. As this is accepted in traditional description, it will be used uncorrected.

In the old face the insertion points of the ligaments and septa are not at the same latitude as their origin; attenuation lengthening results in insertion descending well below in latitude than their deep origin as seen in Figs. 4.5a, b and 4.6.

Electronic Supplementary Material The online version of this chapter (doi:10.1007/978-3-319-69090-2_4) contains supplementary material, which is available to authorized users.

L.C.Y. Ho et al., *The Congruent Facelift*,
https://doi.org/10.1007/978-3-319-69090-2_4

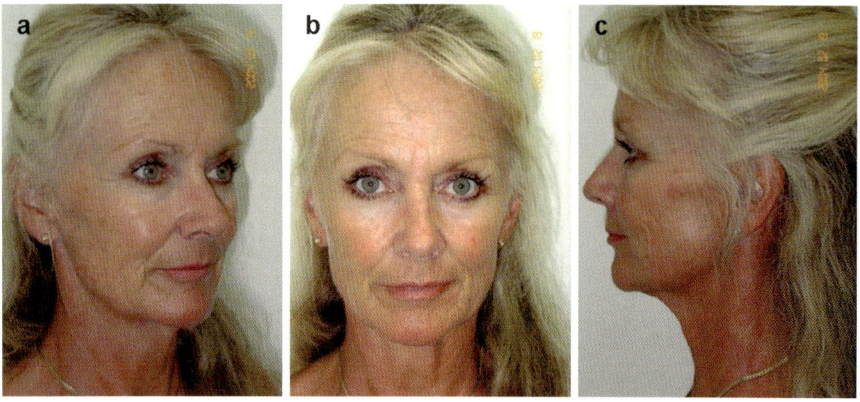

Fig. 4.1 (**a**–**c**) Age stigma

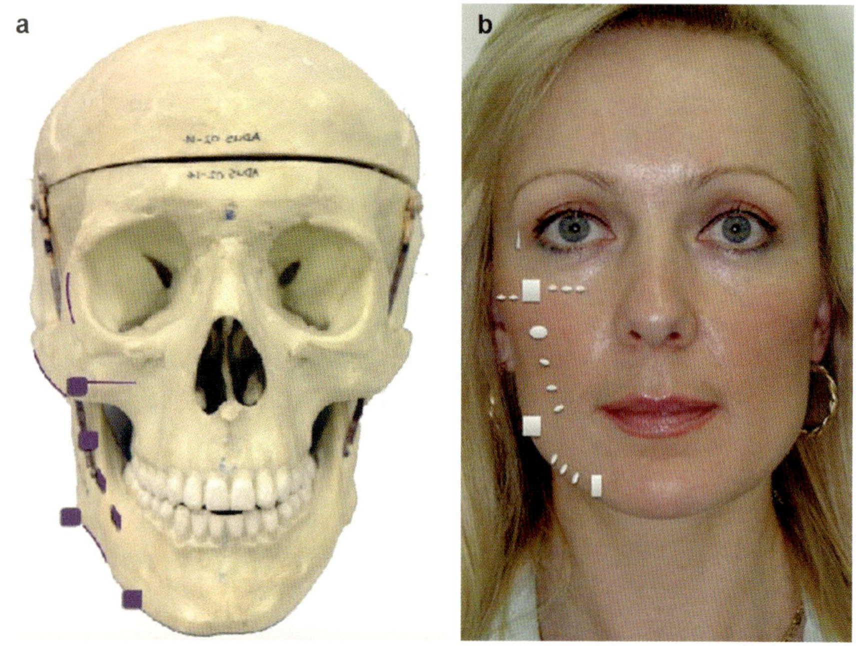

Fig. 4.2 (**a**, **b**) Ligament/septa support system of mid-/lower face

Fat compartment de-voluming and ligament septa attenuation set in motion ptotic gravitation migration of fat compartments along predetermined channels of the weakened system of support generating the well-recognised stigma pattern of eyelid-upper cheek sulcus, nasolabial fold, marionette deformity, jowl and anterior neck bands as demonstrated in graphics in Fig. 4.6 and its reversal in Figs. 4.7a, b. Grey arrowheads indicate directional plane vector for ageing, while green arrowheads indicate required vector in face-lifting to correct these stigmas.

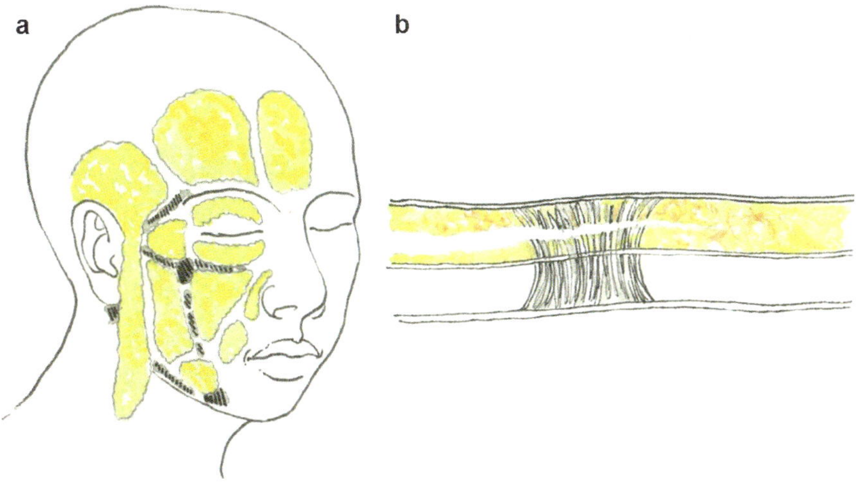

Fig. 4.3 (**a**) Fat compartments in face (**b**) Section showing fat packing and ligament

Fig. 4.4 Face fat compartments structure (Video 4.1)

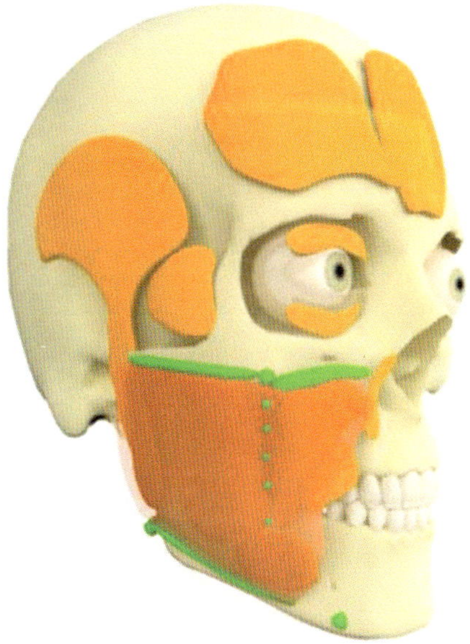

Fat compartment de-voluming together with ligament septa attenuation lengthening leads to lowering the level of both upper and lower horizontal "curtain rods". These lead to changes lower down in the neck and face/neck interphase.

The old neck sags with redundant skin and fat with the stigma troika of anterior neckbands, obtuse cervical-mental angle and an apparently short thicker neck in Fig. 4.8a, b.

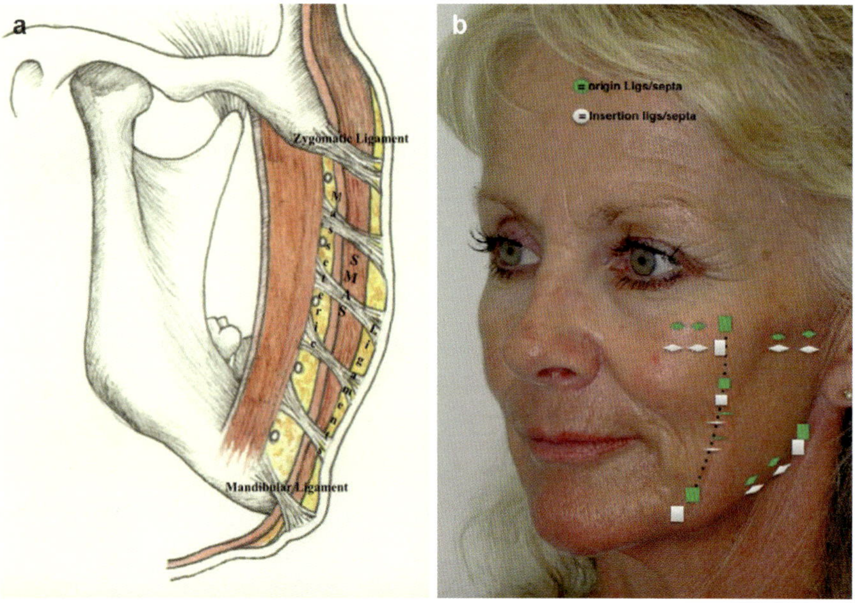

Fig. 4.5 (**a**, **b**) Ligament and septa attenuation and lengthening (Video 4.2)

Fig. 4.6 Compartments de-volume/ ligaments descend (Video 4.3)

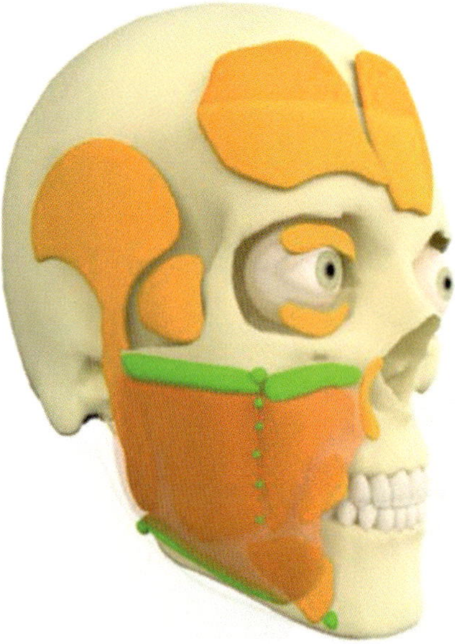

Lowering the lower horizontal curtain rod of mandibular ligament, septa and platysma- auricular ligament system shortens the platysma, which widens to keep its volume constant. As it is adherent to the sternocleidomastoid muscle posteriorly, it pushes its anterior ventral border forwards. This widening effect is augmented by ageing hypertonicity (Fig. 4.9 Andreas Vesalius) of this

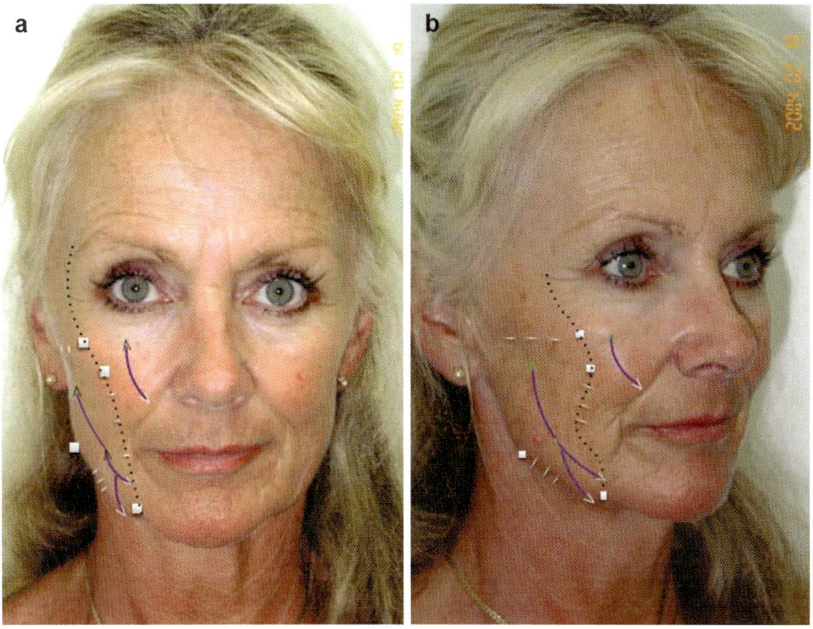

Fig. 4.7 (**a**, **b**) Ptotic gravitational migration fat compartments and skin. Grey arrowheads indicate directional plane vector for ageing, while green arrowheads indicate required vector in face-lifting to correct these stigmas

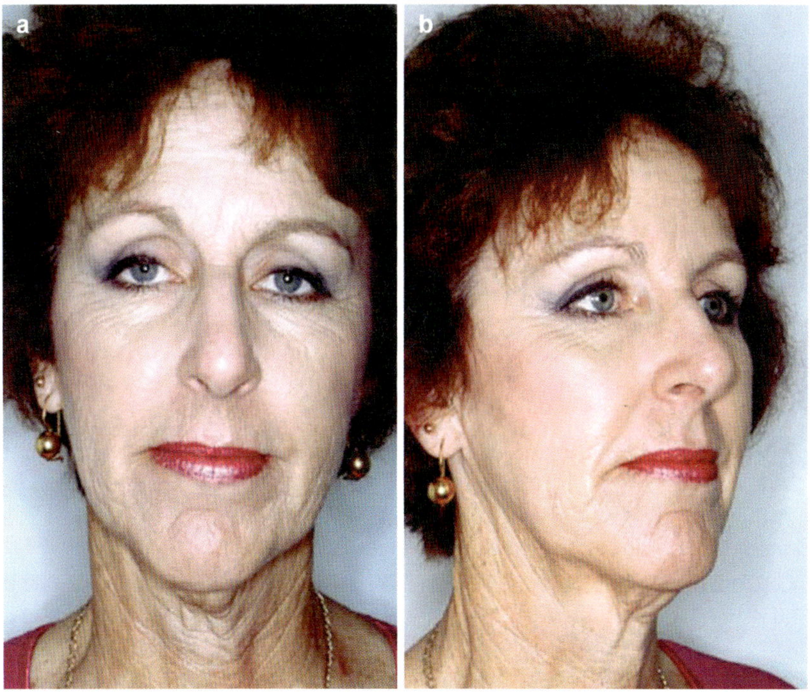

Fig. 4.8 (**a**, **b**) Aged neck stigma

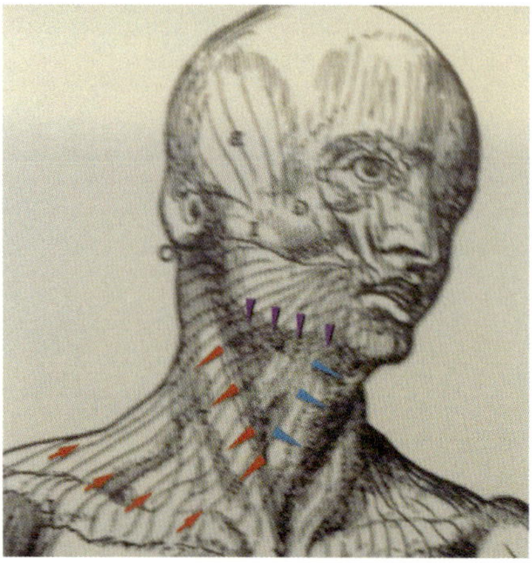

Fig. 4.9 Andreas Vesalius on platysma/SMAS (Courtesy Jeremy Norman & Co., Inc.)

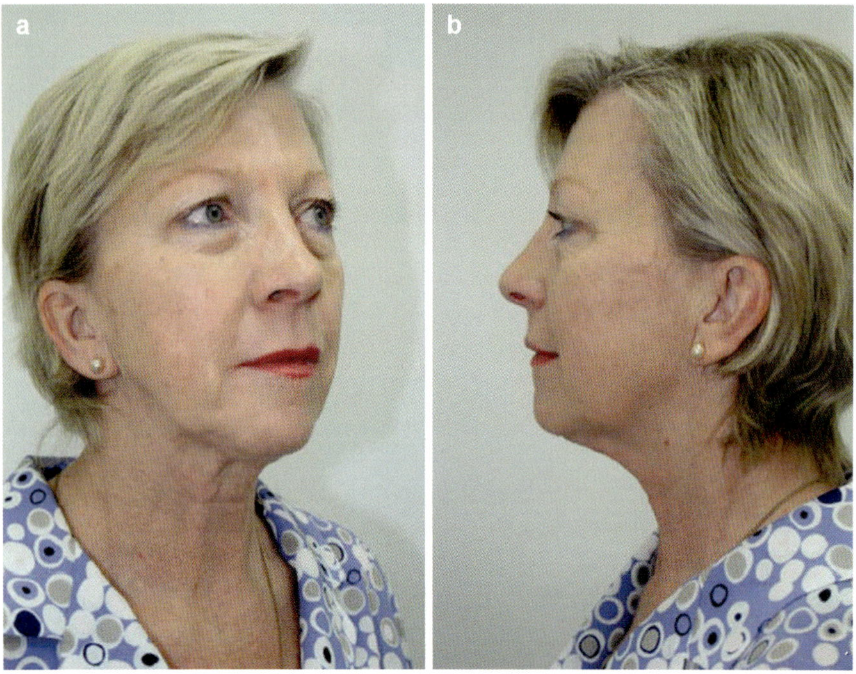

Fig. 4.10 (**a**, **b**) Neck bands and obtuse angle neck

preeminent muscle of facial expression. This protruding muscle border is an expression band, much like the frown lines and crow's feet.

The local intrinsic causes of the obtuse cervical-mental angle are the progressive increase in size of the inverted "L"-shaped platysma band, lax submental skin and fat and enlarged deep para-hyoid fat pad (Figs. 4.10a, b and 4.11).

Fig. 4.11 Para-hyoid fat pad

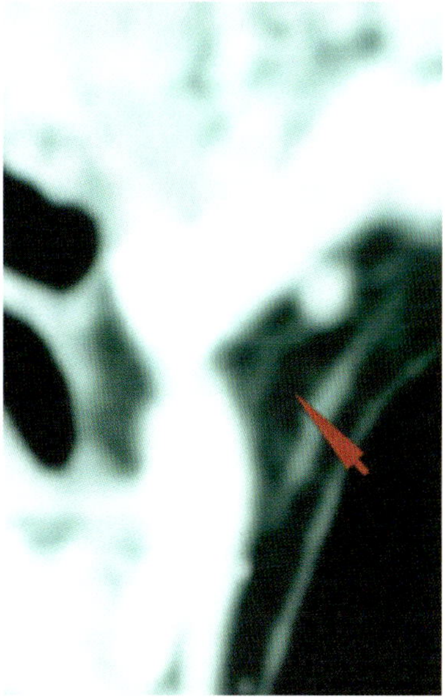

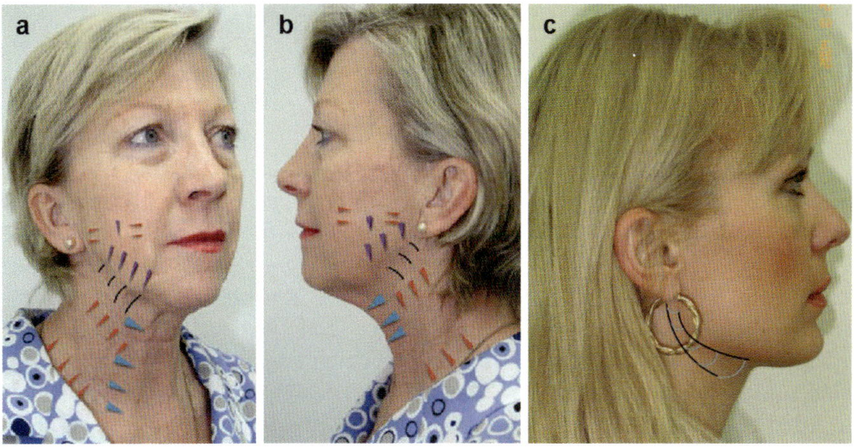

Fig. 4.12 (**a–c**) Face/neck interphase

Extrinsic causes are the descent of the mandibular ligament/septa and platysma- auricular ligament "curtain rod" and the "herniating jowl" pushing the posterior submental triangle caudally.

The thick short neck is the last and final unattractive stigma of the ageing neck. Its girth is increased by the development of the anterior platysma band and excess fat growth and accumulation at the upper end of the neck cylinder. Its apparent height is shortened by the development of the anterior platysma band and the descent of the jowl.

The face neck interphase is the area of the submandibular triangles at the side and the submental triangle in front (Fig. 4.12a, b). It is bordered above by

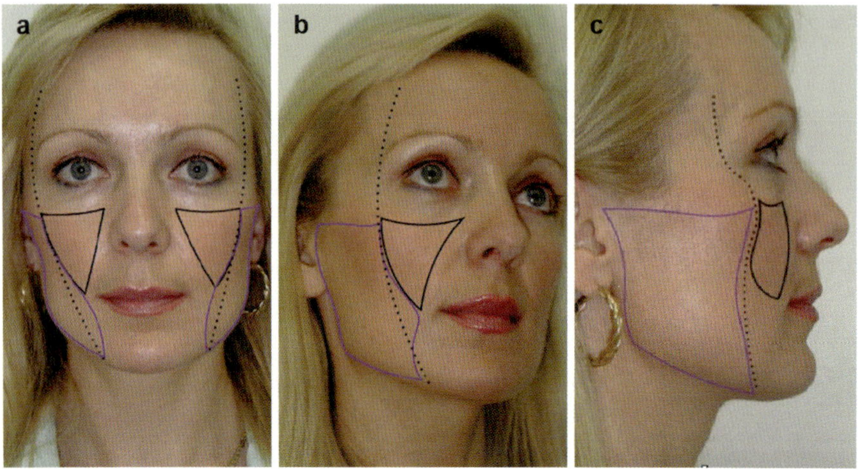

Fig. 4.13 (a–c) Three-dimensional contour face, face planes and sub-planes

the mandibular margin and inferiorly by the anterior belly of the digastric muscle and the hyoid bone and posteriorly by the posterior belly of the digastric to the mandibular angle/upper sternocleidomastoid gutter.

Its floor is the local part of the platysma muscle. Age hypertonicity causes tenting of this muscular floor with loss of the delicate concave contour below the mandibular margin seen in Fig. 4.12c.

The sum of the stigmas in this important but so far largely neglected region is its intrinsic stigma plus those visited on it from the descending face above and the rest of the neck below; these stigmas are correctable with a coherent congruent approach.

An effective face-lift must address the issues of the three-dimensional contour of the face and neck (Fig. 4.13a–c) and their interphase junction in addition to the plane changeover junction where the lower half of the outer face effectively appears prominently in both front and side planes with changing shapes on face rotation (Fig. 4.13a–c). Effective recompression/recontouring of sagging decompressed compartment soft tissue/fat and their containment ligaments and septa with congruent contour enforcement loops and plane congruent vector forces securing them firmly at the proper youthful latitude will deliver an optimum natural-looking lasting result.

4.2 Congruent Face-Lift Surgical Procedure

4.2.1 Preoperative Preparation

Anaesthesia

The congruent face-lift is performed under facial nerve blocks and neuroleptic anaesthesia with an anaesthetist in attendance. Healthy patients with no significant co-morbidity may be discharged the same day; others may have to stay overnight as indicated.

Preoperative Marking for Congruent Face-Lift
This is performed (Fig. 4.14) pre-sedation with the patient in the erect posture standing or sitting to plan the skin incisions, skin excision, novel L Ho dermal pennant flaps, limits of dissection (and plane changeover junction as required).

4.2.2 Steps of Operation

The patient is suitably positioned on the operating table. After initial sedation and blocks to the infraorbital, mental and preauricular nerves and the cervical plexus, subcutaneous hydrodissection is commenced by injection of 30 ml Fournier's mix on each side in the subcutaneous plane of each temple, cheek, submentum and upper neck. Fournier's mix is injected into the upper mid neck for liposuction here. Submental liposuction is performed first with syringe and cannula. Particular attention is paid to the para-hyoid fat deep to the cervical fascia as this is essential to produce a good cervical-mental angle and clear definition of the bilateral isosceles and submandibular triangles. Care should be exercised when liposuction is performed out in the lateral regions when required as the neck in these elderly patients often suffers from carotid atherosclerosis. The vertically inverted "L" incision is made, and the proposed dermal pennant flaps are incised and de-epithelialised (Figs. 4.15a, b and 4.16). The cephalic dermal flap is designed about 10 mm below the helical root and the caudal one below the earlobe.

The precise amount of skin removed is dictated by the estimated amount of skin redundancy to be excised; this is significantly less than Joseph's excision as it is not just skin only "lift". The lateral cheek skin is undermined in the subcutaneous plane over the SMAS/platysma layer splitting the subcutaneous fat horizontally evenly by

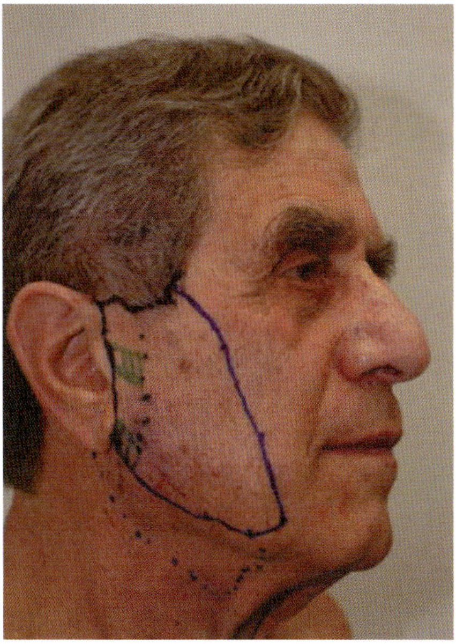

Fig. 4.14 Preoperative markings

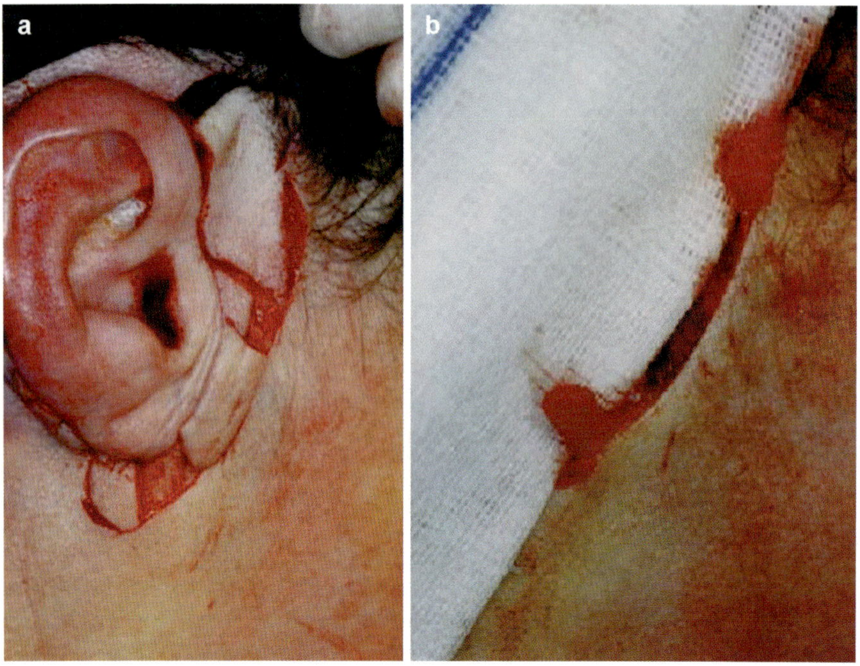

Fig. 4.15 (**a**) Incisions (**b**) Dermal pennant flaps

Fig. 4.16 Subcutaneous dissection

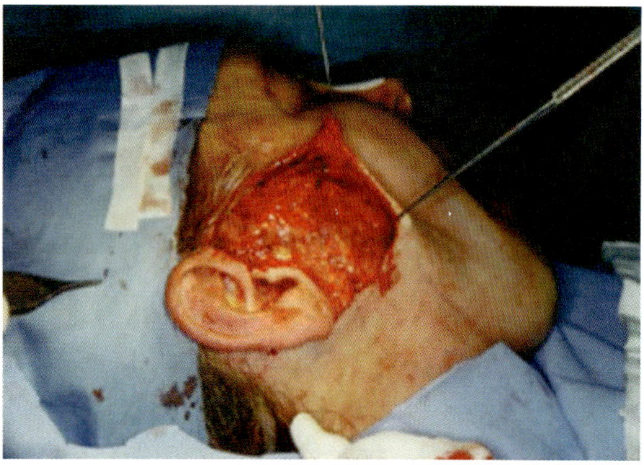

sharp (Fig. 4.3b) dissection initially and then with a moist saline gauze swab towards the plane changeover junction (Fig. 4.17a–c). The dissection is carried out to the zygomatic ligament and maxillary buccal septa superiorly and the masseter ligament/septa medially. These are preserved. The mandibular and platysma-auricular ligaments are preserved. The mandibular septa are sectioned and dissection extended into the neck to the level of the hyoid bone when skin excess is moderate or severe and platysma bands are prominent. Haemostasis is carried out along the way.

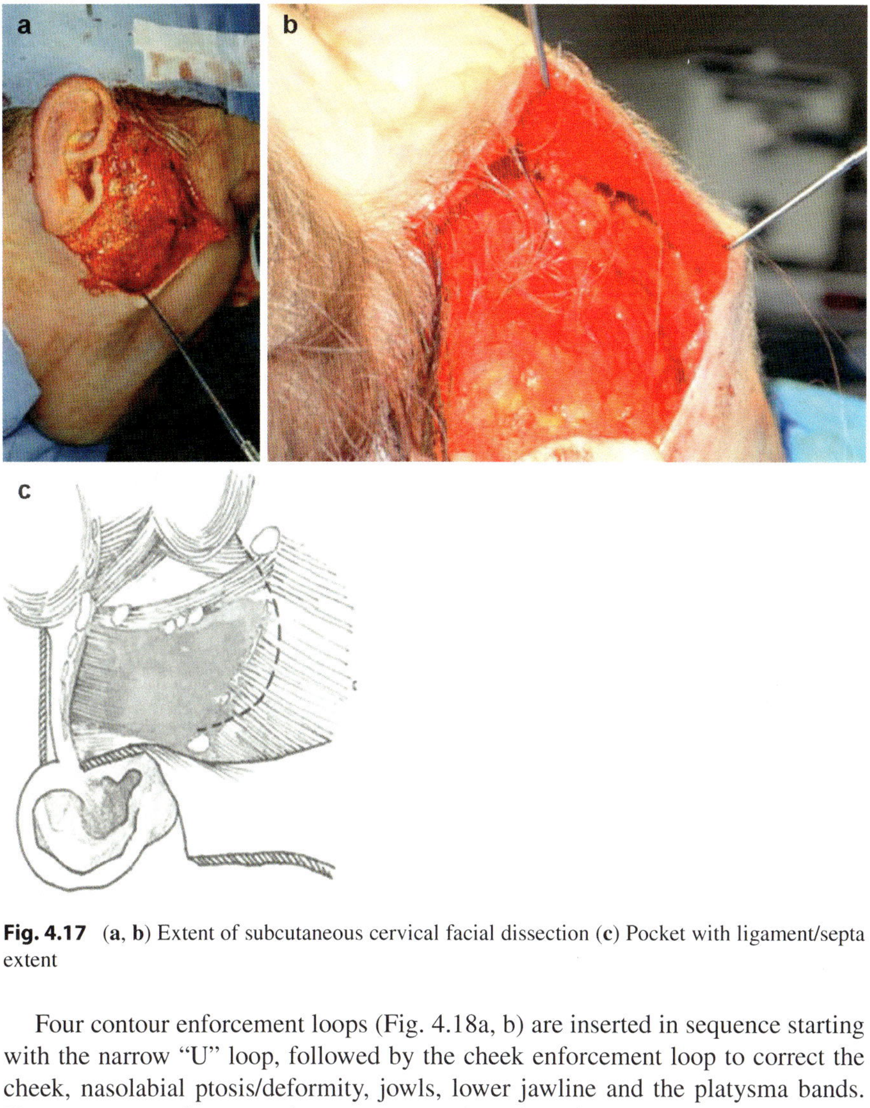

Fig. 4.17 (**a**, **b**) Extent of subcutaneous cervical facial dissection (**c**) Pocket with ligament/septa extent

Four contour enforcement loops (Fig. 4.18a, b) are inserted in sequence starting with the narrow "U" loop, followed by the cheek enforcement loop to correct the cheek, nasolabial ptosis/deformity, jowls, lower jawline and the platysma bands. These contour enforcement loops are woven into the reticular portion of the osseous and deep fascia cutaneous ligaments and septa at their junction through the SMAS [2]. When tightened and secured, they act as tight guy ropes and compress the relevant fat compartments, elevating the ptosed facial soft tissue compartments into their original youthful latitude. The first three are anchored firmly above the zygomatic arch into the strong temporal fascia, while the fourth secures the platysma band firmly to the mastoid fascia.

A long narrow "U"-shaped purse string ("G") suture loop (Fig. 4.19a, b) runs from just above the zygomatic arch in front of the preauricular incision line to the mandibular angle taking in the platysma-auricular ligament and back up. This is tightened optimally and secured to the temporal fascia.

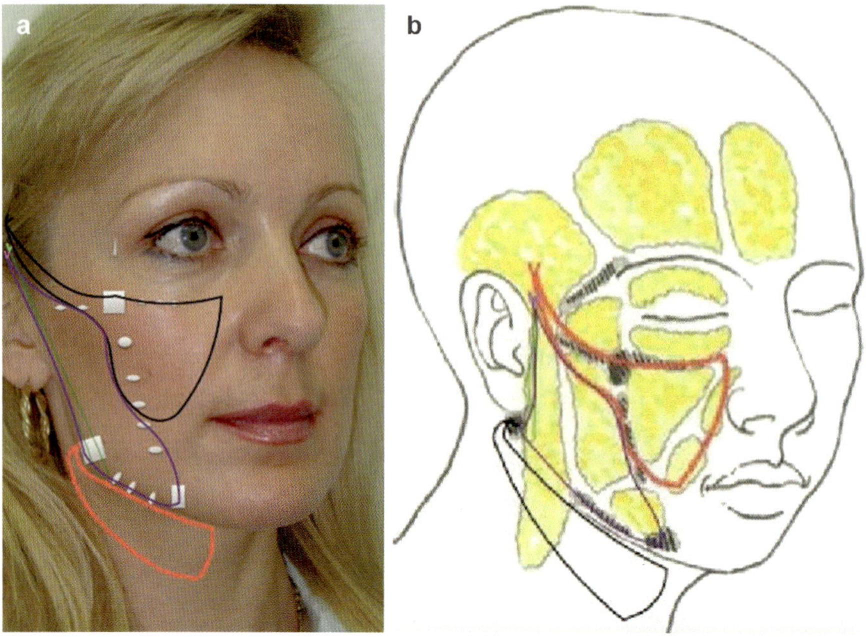

Fig. 4.18 (**a**, **b**) Four contour enforcement loops

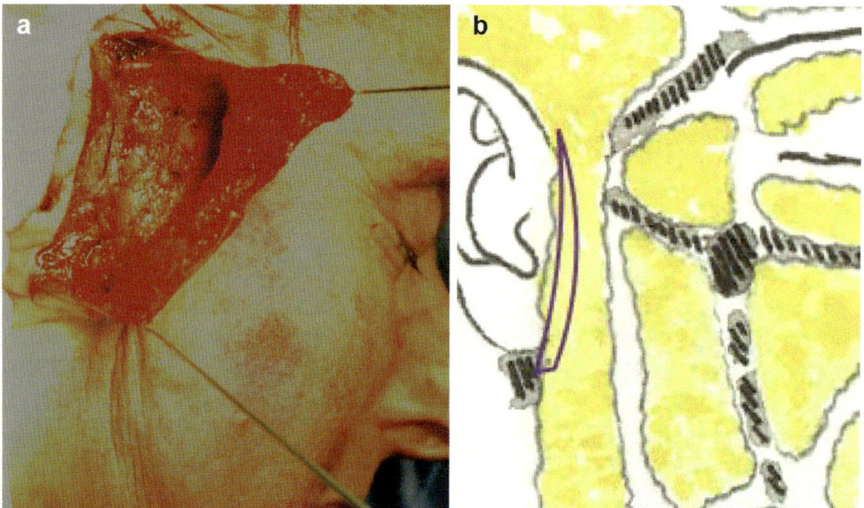

Fig. 4.19 (**a**, **b**) Narrow U loop

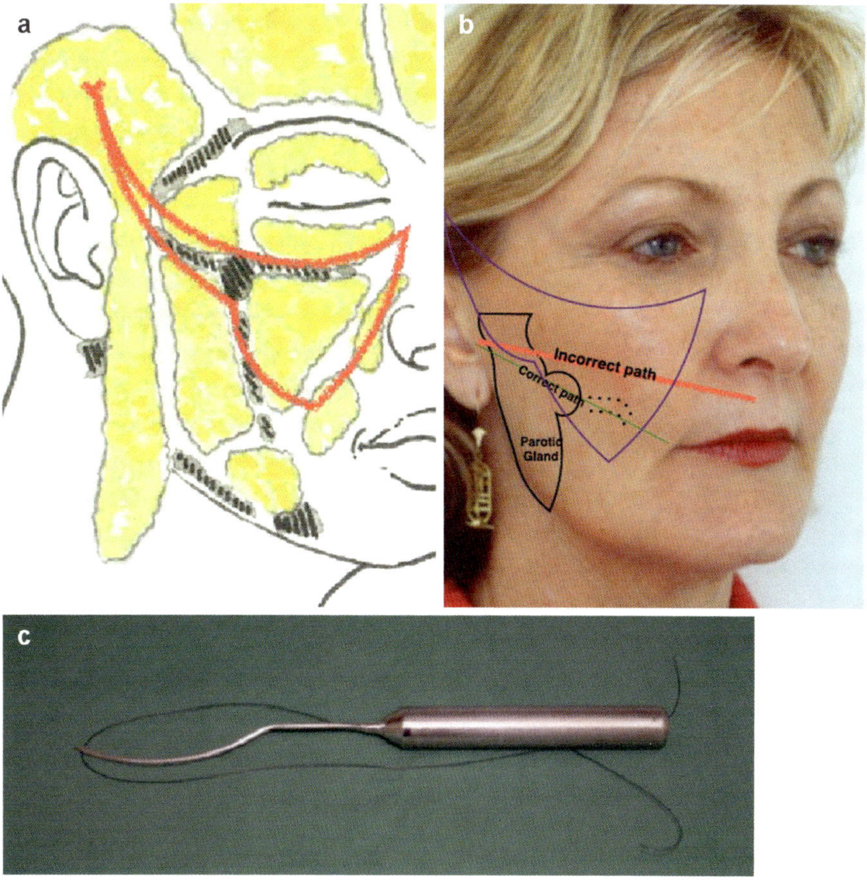

Fig. 4.20 (**a**, **b**) Extent of cheek contour enforcement loop (**c**) L Ho cheek enforce needle from austramedex.com

The 2.0 Prolene cheek loop (Figs. 4.20a, b) is sutured securely to the temporal fascia above. Insertion of the loop is made easy with the L Ho needle Fig. 4.20c. The parotid duct is clear of the track of this loop.

Insertion starts at the top through a small stab incision above the horizontal limb of the preauricular incision, manoeuvring it down and forward through the zygomatic ligament and then the overlying skin (Fig. 4.21a–d).

The needle is unthreaded, removed through the temporal incision and rethreaded at the malar puncture wound. It is then reinserted here and manoeuvred around the upper and medial cheek margins to emerge through a puncture wound in the oral mucosa in front of the second molar tooth (Figs. 4.22a–d and 4.23a–d).

It is then unthreaded and the needle is removed from mucosal puncture wound and rethreaded within the mouth and reinserted through the buccal mucosal wound to emerge in the soft tissue under the cervical facial flap at the vertical dropped from the zygomatic ligament.

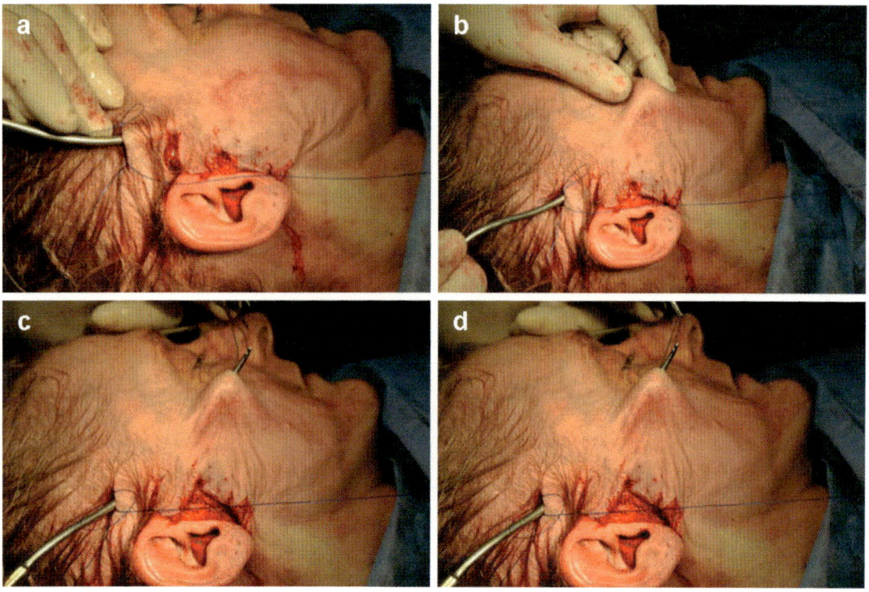

Fig. 4.21 (**a**, **b**) Insertion of temporal segment of cheek loop. (**c**, **d**) Unthreading of needle prior to reinsertion for a 90° change of direction

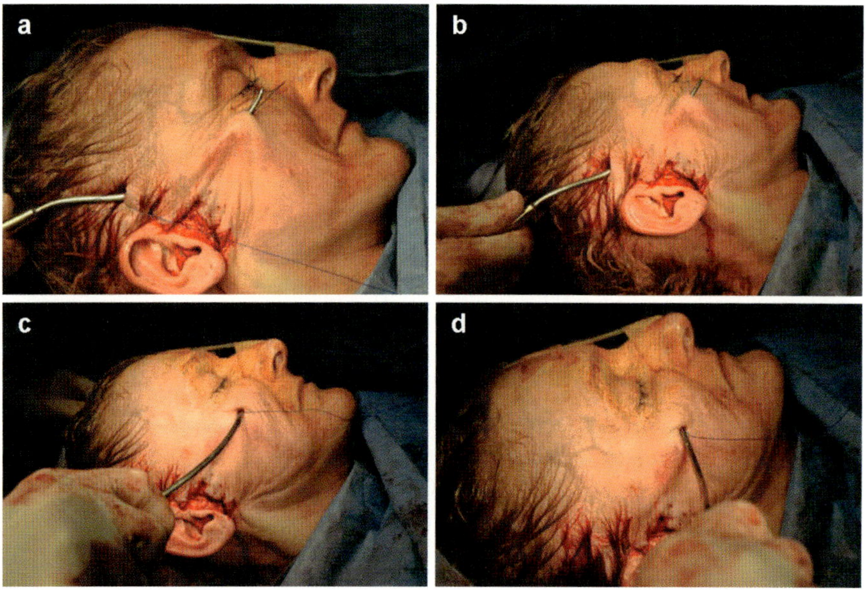

Fig. 4.22 (**a**–**d**) Percutaneous unthreading and rethreading of suture and reinsertion

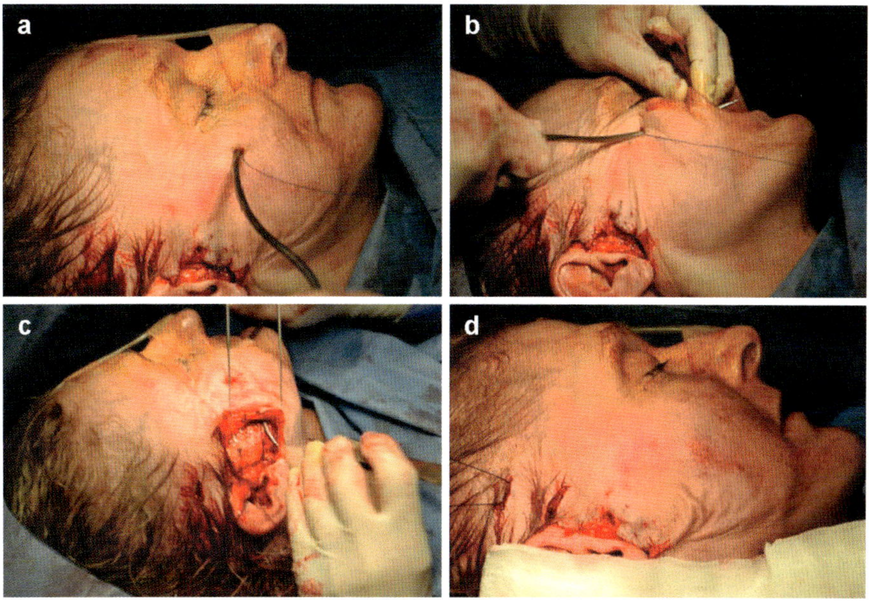

Fig. 4.23 (**a–d**) Needle exteriorised, unthreaded, rethreaded, reinserted; this repeated till the upper temporal incision is reached

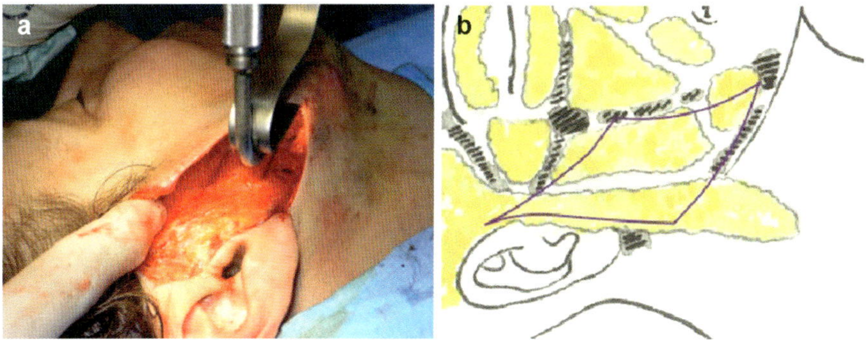

Fig. 4.24 (**a**, **b**) Rhomboid loop insertion

The previously described unthreading, withdrawal of needle, rethreading and reinserting and manoeuvring are repeated thrice till the suture loop reaches the short temporal incision where it is optimally tightened and secured in the strong temporal fascia.

The third loop is the rhomboid-shaped enforcement suture loop starting in the temporal fascia above the zygomatic arch picking up the SMAS/platysma fascia aponeurotic system bounded laterally by the ramus of the mandible, the lower mandibular margin back up along the oral masseteric and lateral cheek pilasters and up above the zygomatic arch to be securely tightened (Fig. 4.24a, b) to the temporal fascia.

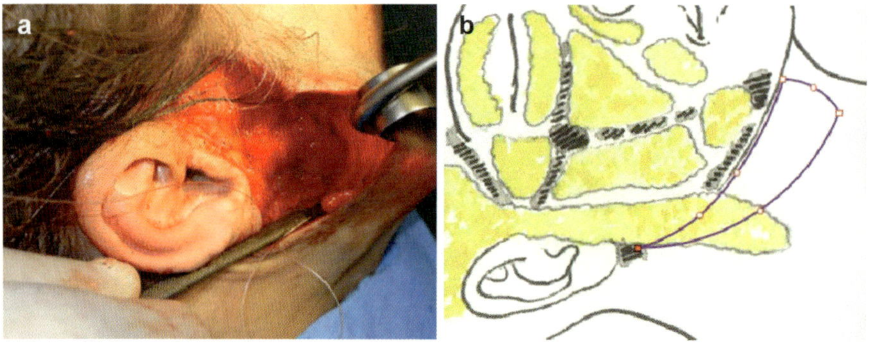

Fig. 4.25 (**a**, **b**) Contour enforcement loop for anterior platysma band

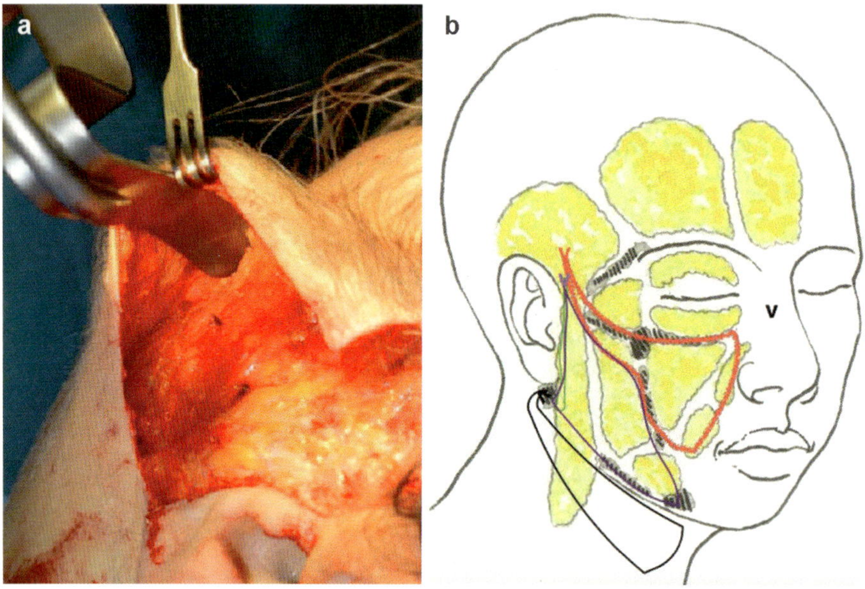

Fig. 4.26 (**a**, **b**) Completion of four contour enforcement loop insertion

The prominent anterior platysma border is corrected by a long triangular enforcement loop tightened and securely fixed deeply to the mastoid fascia. It starts in the mastoid fascia behind the mastoid tip running below the mandibular margin, then just behind the border of the upper platysma band for 2.5 cm and then back to the mastoid tip to be tied securely to (Fig. 4.25a, b) its fascia. The suture tension is controlled by the slip knot technique which allows precision and symmetrical congruent tightening of the superficial fascia system of the face. Finally after all four loops (Fig. 4.26a, b) have been inserted, excess skin is estimated and trimmed off with cephalic vector in mind.

The skin is re-draped with a predominantly cephalic vector and trimmed. The lower dermal pennant flap is positioned and sutured to the mastoid fascia through a tunnel via the earlobe base and a post-auricular stab incision (Fig. 4.27a, b). The

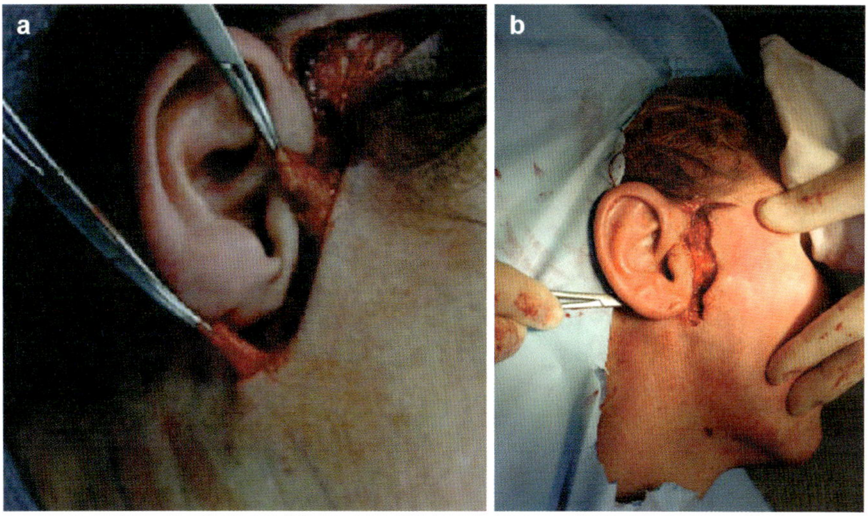

Fig. 4.27 (**a**, **b**) Dermal pennant flaps; inferior flap tunnelled through earlobe

Fig. 4.28 Superior dermal pennant flap fixation

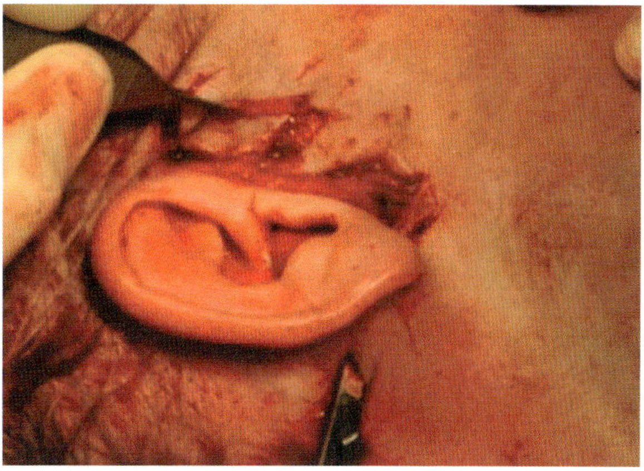

superior flap (Fig. 4.28) is fixed to the temporal fascia above and behind the angle of the incision. Flexibility and final tailoring of this dermal pennant flap are possible and desirable.

The preauricular skin wounds are then closed tension-free (Fig. 4.29a–d) with the novel L Ho trans-cartilaginous horizontal mattress sutures. The face and neck are thoroughly cleaned and dried (Fig. 4.29e). The suture lines are steristriped and an appropriate head dressing is applied. The patient is discharged later in the day when fit or may stay overnight. Sutures are removed 10 days post-operatively.

The reconstructive procedure has been designed to move and secure the ligaments and septa's insertion points to the youthful latitude with simultaneous recompression and recontouring of the soft tissue/fat compartments. These actions are shown in Figs. 4.30 and 4.31 in front and oblique views in five steps.

The goal of rejuvenation facial aesthetic surgery is to produce a youthful, firm, full and "non-dropped" face with youthfully positioned clean-cut well-defined features and

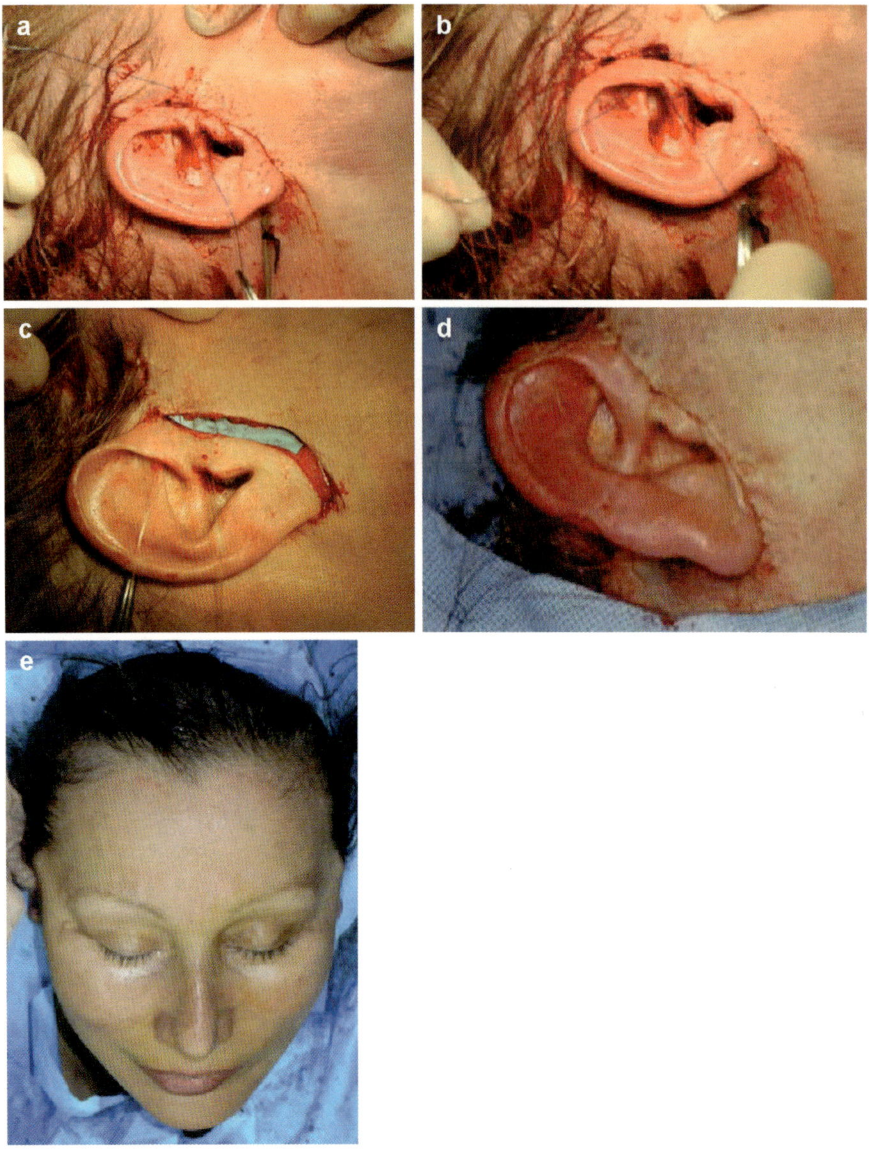

Fig. 4.29 (**a**, **b**) Closure with L Ho trans-cartilaginous horizontal mattress sutures. (**c**, **d**) Completion of L Ho trans-cartilaginous suture. (**e**) Face/neck cleaned

margins in the face. The convex nature of the changeover junction of lateral and front planes of the mid- and lower face and the concave nature of the changeover junction of the mandibular border/upper neck interphase should be preserved and refined in face-lift surgery. Failure to do so may result in an unnatural-looking face and neck. The

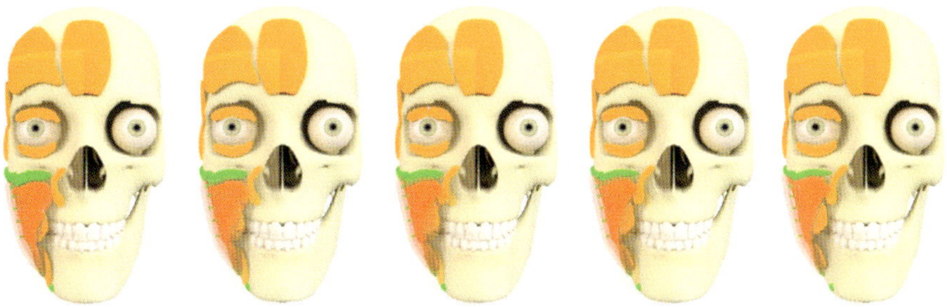

Fig. 4.30 Sequential tightening loops in front view (Video 4.4)

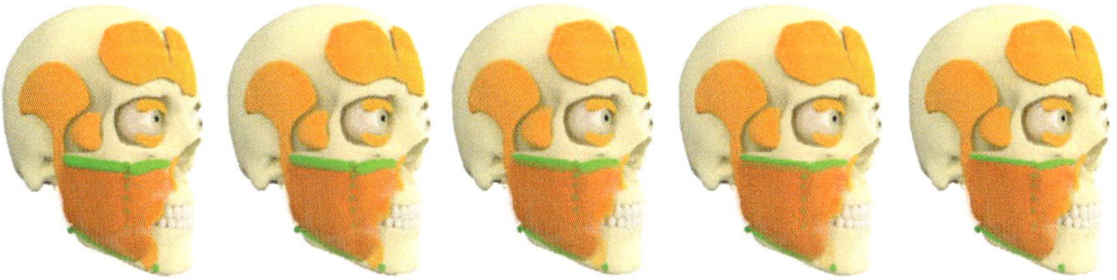

Fig. 4.31 Sequential tightening loops in oblique view (Video 4.5)

lower face will have a broad flat appearance; the mandibular border will be irregular and fuzzy and the angle lacking a chiselled natural prominence.

4.2.3 Case Studies

Eight case studies with eight very different ageing patient types who have undergone the procedure are shown in Figs. 4.32a–c, 4.33, 4.34, 4.35, 4.36, 4.37, 4.38 and 4.39a–c. A critical look at the after images will allow the reader to pick up shortfalls in the operative technique of the senior surgeon author in the execution of the precision required in loop suture insertion and optimum tension required in tightening the contour enforcement loops to prevent feature "deformities" and enhance the youthful features and contour. An optimum long-lasting result requires optimum nondeforming tension to tighten these enforcement loops and precise skin excision with a cephalic vector in the appropriate plane of the face. This requires good clinical judgement and experience. Figure 4.40a–d shows quality of the preauricular scars.

Five case studies with three morphed smiling views from before to last follow-up are shown in Figs. 4.41a–c, 4.42, 4.43, 4.44 and 4.45a–c. These demonstrate the rejuvenated soft youthful smile is a function of the congruently youthful repositioned muscle excursion. Likewise, aged mimesis and smile are due to progressive caudally displaced mimetic muscle excursion.

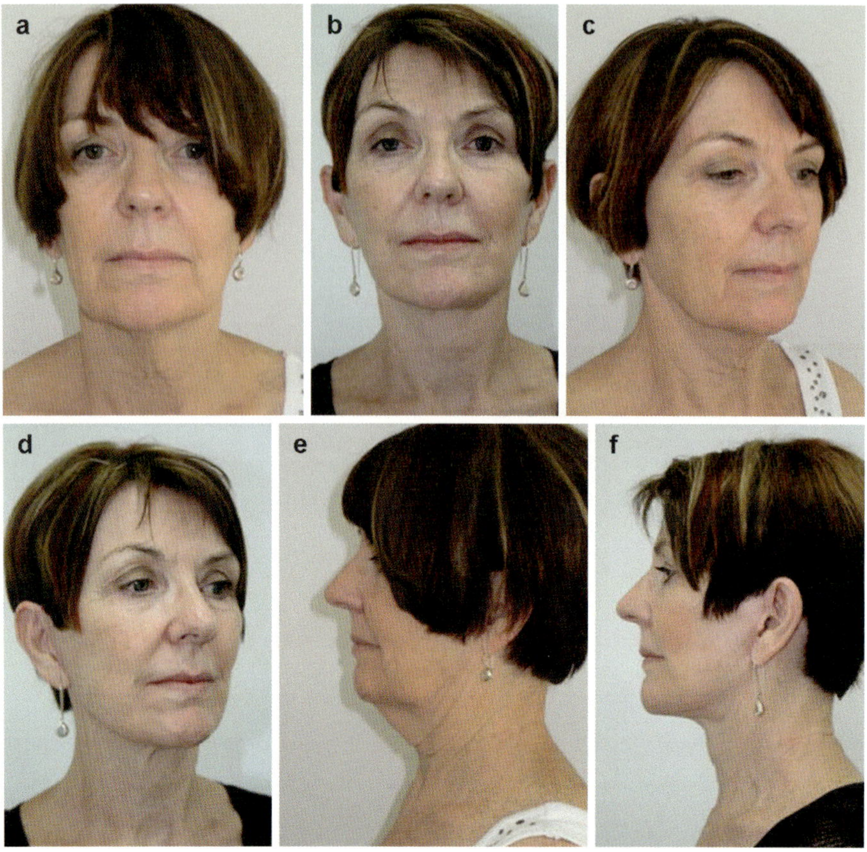

Fig. 4.32 Patient SH, age 57. (**a**, **c**, **e**) Before—flat droopy cheeks and jowls, irregular jawline and webbed neck. (**b**, **d**, **f**) Post-operative 3 years (*Adapted from Ho* [18])

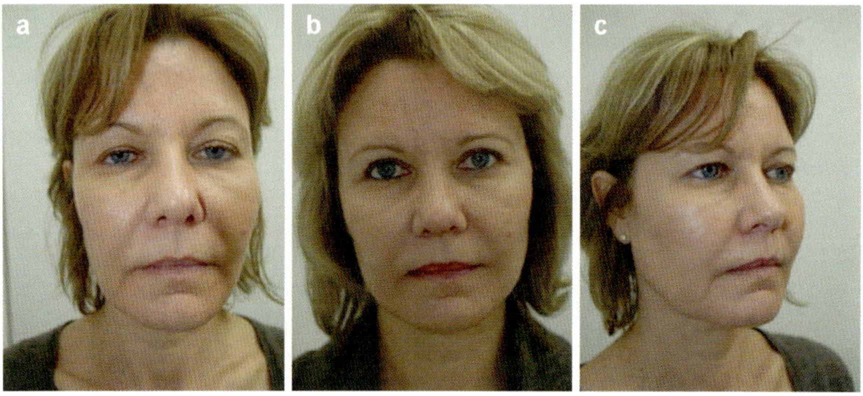

Fig. 4.33 Patient KD, age 47. (**a**, **c**, **e**) Before—flat droopy cheeks, fuzzy jawline and poor cervical-mental angle. (**b**, **d**, **f**) Post-operative 3.5 years (*Adapted from Ho* [18])

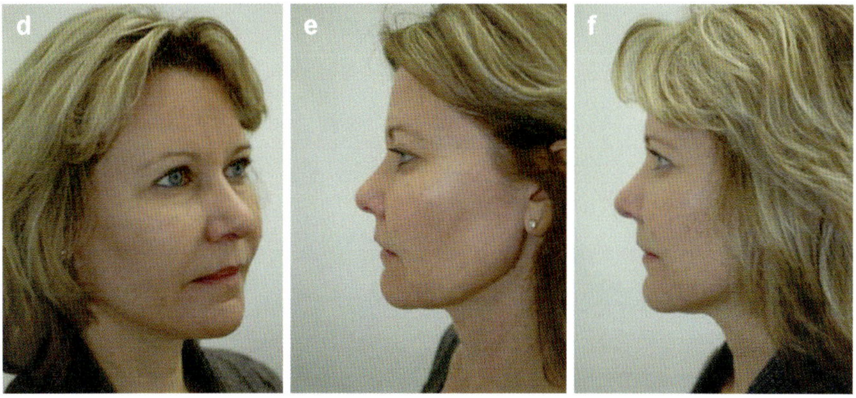

Fig. 4.33 (continued)

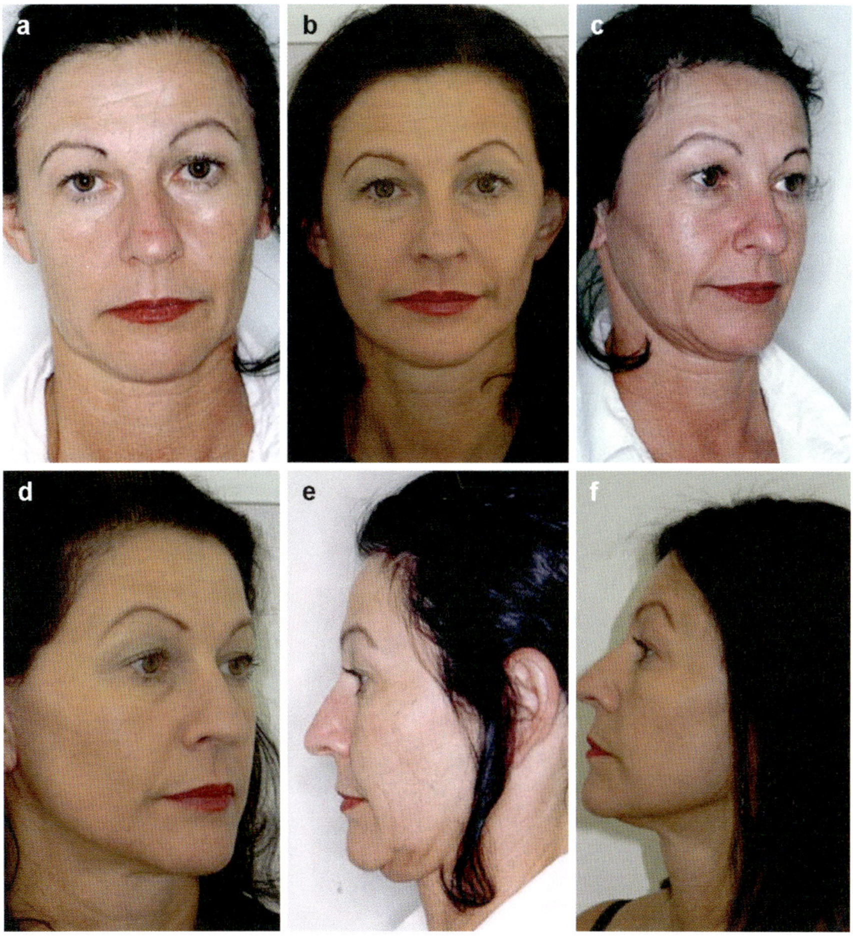

Fig. 4.34 Patient DC, age 45. (**a**, **c**, **e**) Before—large flat droopy cheek, fuzzy jawline poor cervical-mental angle. (**b**, **d**, **f**) Post-operative—2 years post-operative

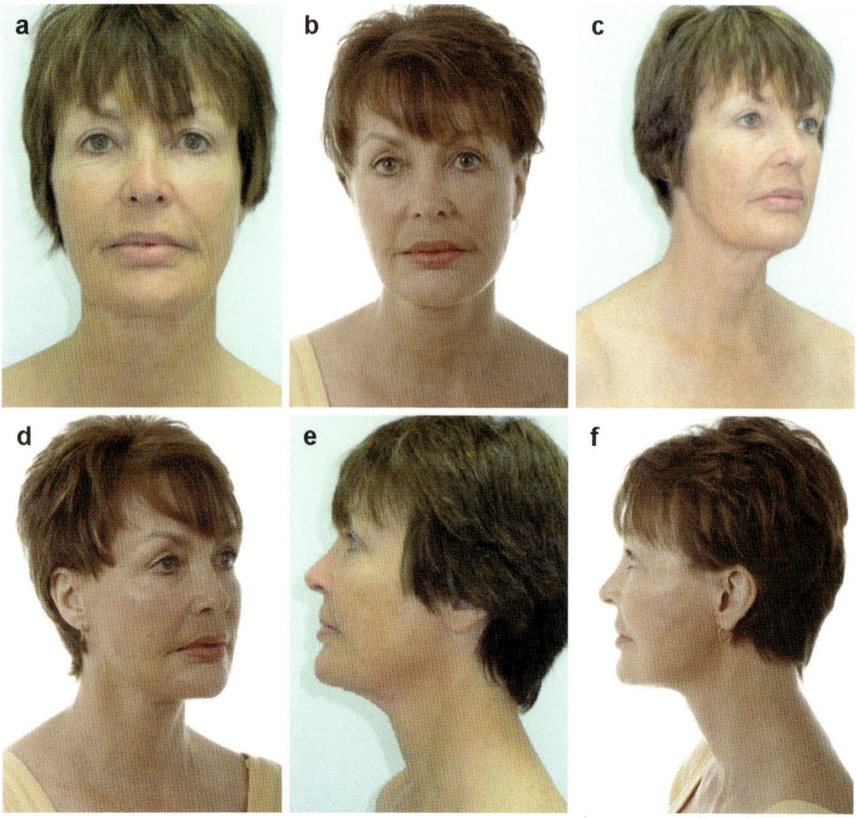

Fig. 4.35 Patient PD, age 57. Previous face-lift 2 years before. (**a**, **c**, **e**) Before—flat cheeks, poor jawline and neck. (**b**, **d**, **f**) Post-operative 2.5 years (*Adapted from Ho* [18])

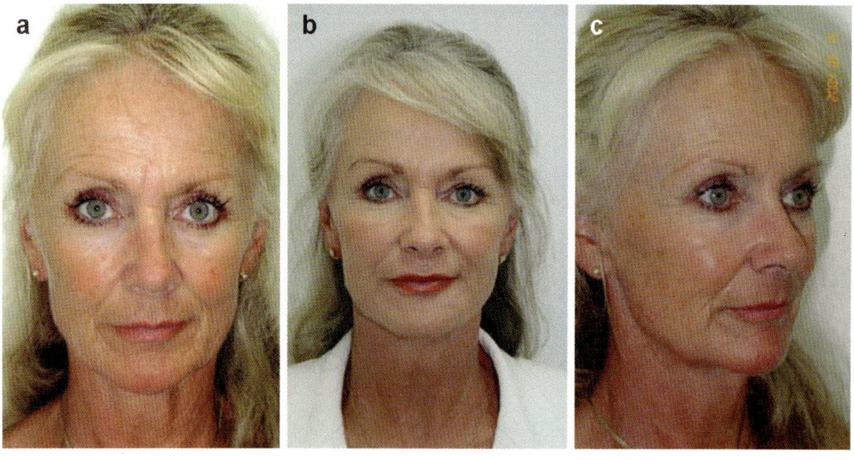

Fig. 4.36 Patient PVC, age 53.(**a**, **c**, **e**) Before—flat cheek and poor cervical-mental angle. (**b**, **d**, **f**) Post-operative 3 years

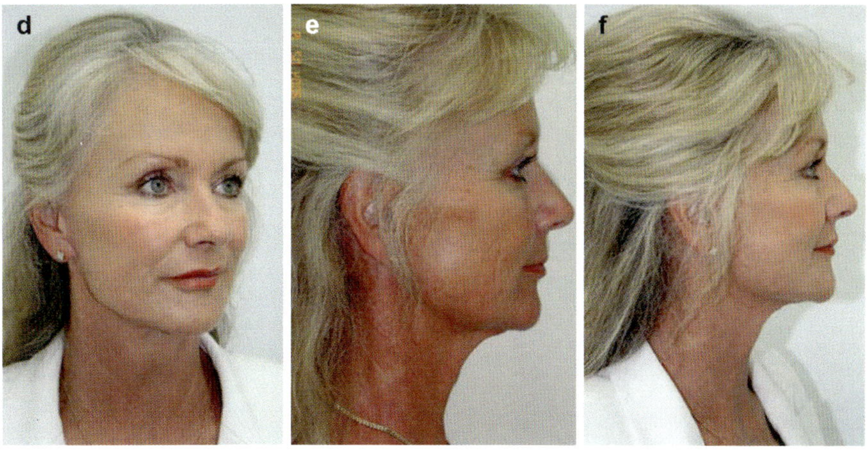

Fig. 4.36 (continued)

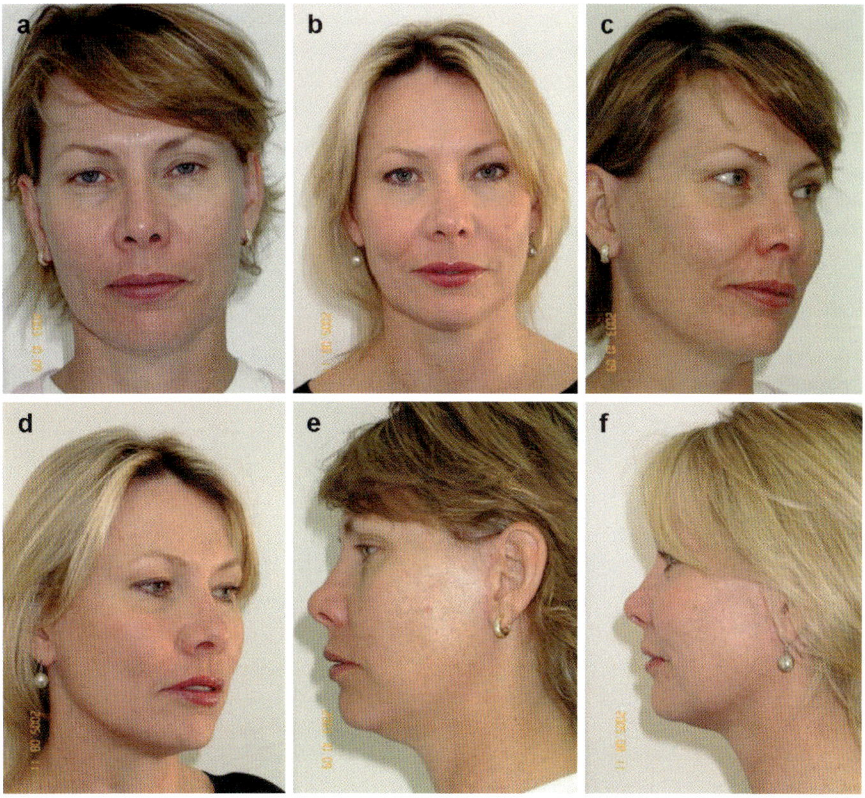

Fig. 4.37 Patient SMH, age 46. (**a**, **c**, **e**) Before—early ageing; flat cheeks, poorly defined jawline and obtuse cervical-mental angle. (**b**, **d**, **f**) Post-operative 4 years

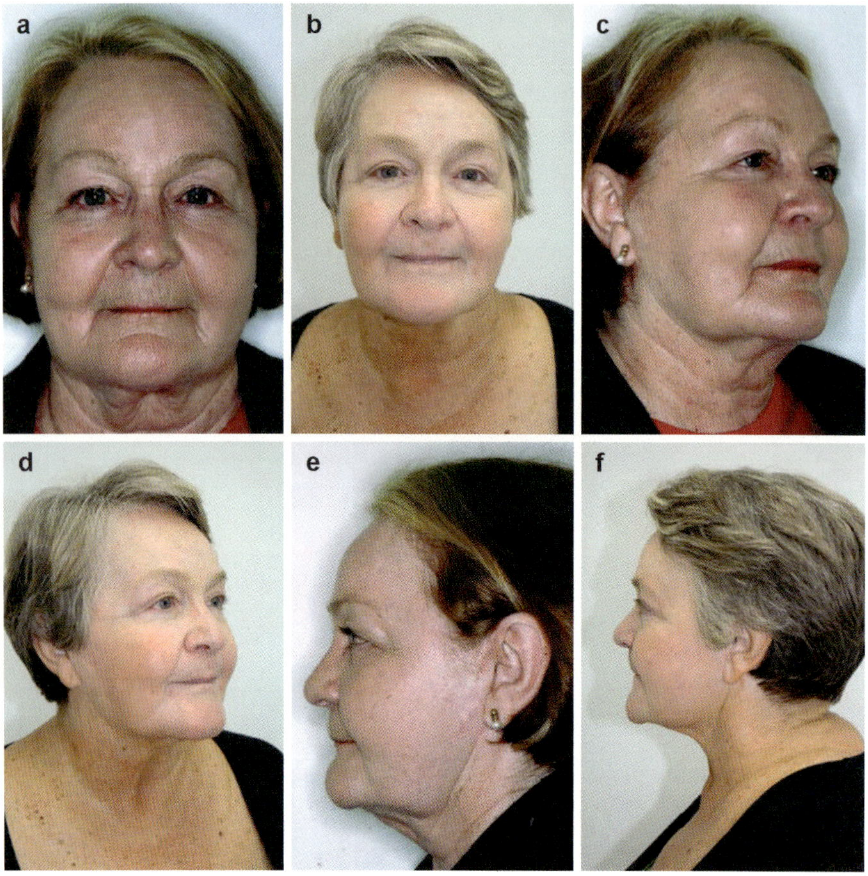

Fig. 4.38 Patient VL, aged 69. Unhappy with previous face-lift a year ago. (**a**, **c**, **e**) Before. (**b**, **d**, **f**) Post-operative 3 years

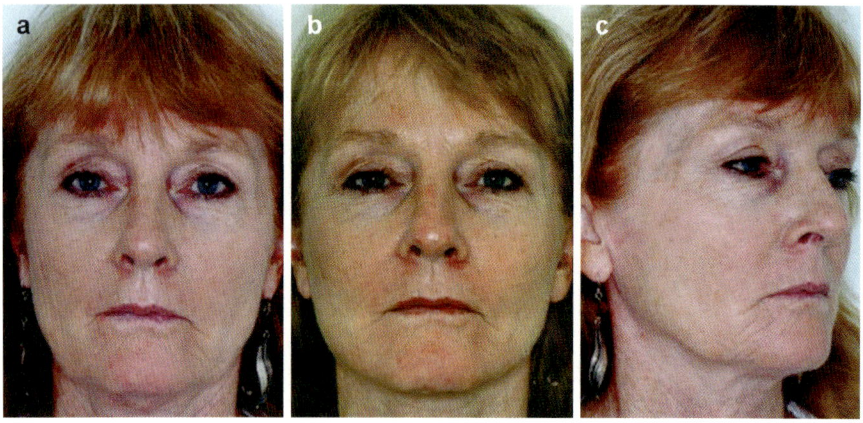

Fig. 4.39 Patient RS, aged 63. (**a**, **c**, **e**) Before—severe sun damage and heavy wrinkle and expression lines. (**b**, **d**, **f**) Post-operative 3.5 years

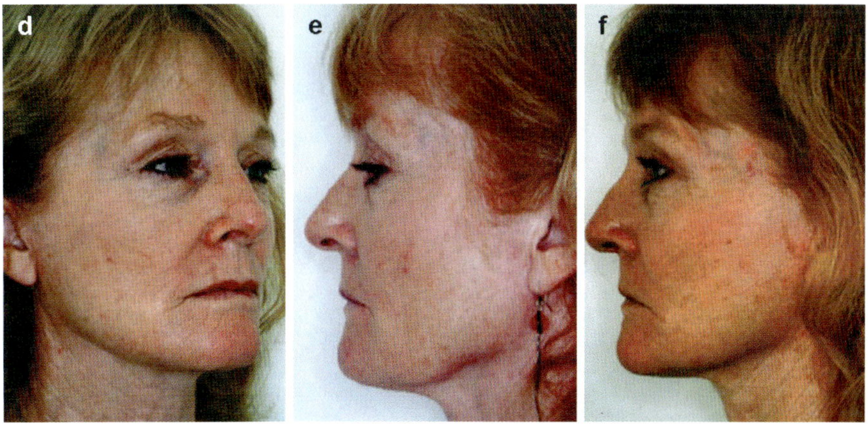

Fig. 4.39 (continued)

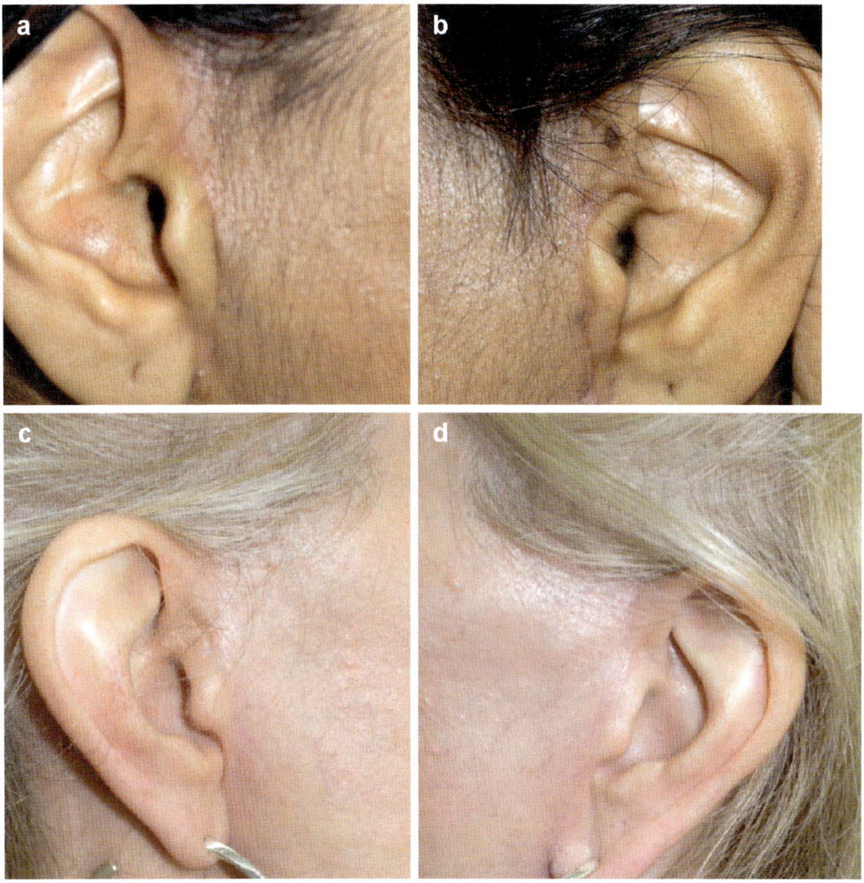

Fig. 4.40 (**a**–**d**) Post-operative preauricular scars

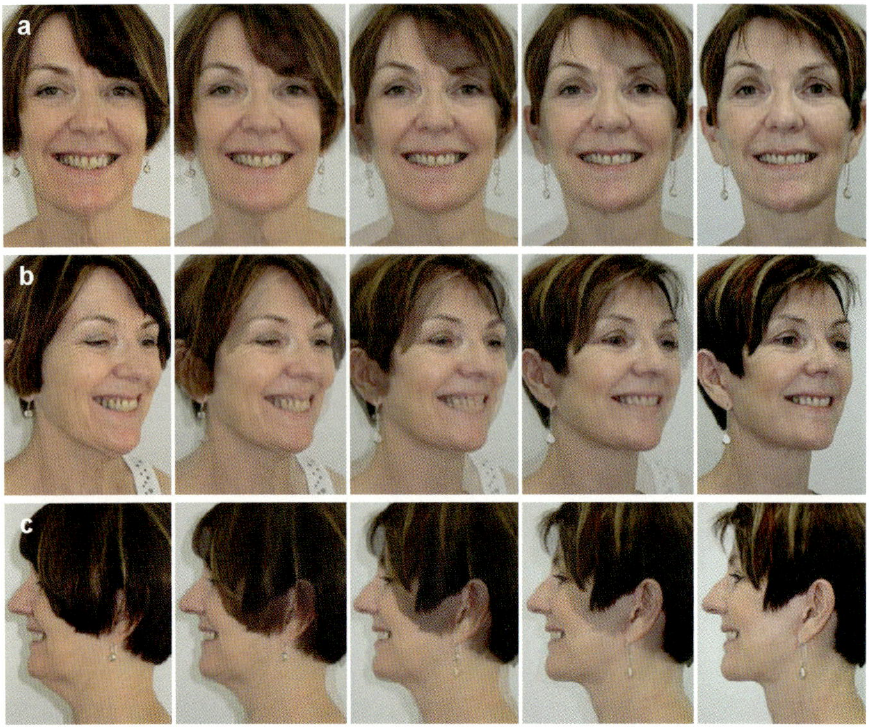

Fig. 4.41 (**a**–**c**) Patient SH. The face-lift of SH is morphed in a series of five sequential morphing changes from preoperative to 3 years post-operative

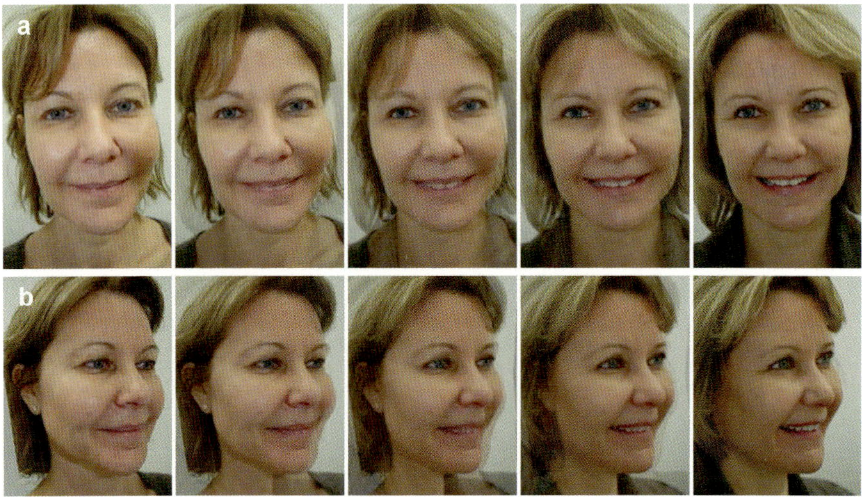

Fig. 4.42 (**a**–**c**) Patient KED. The face-lift of KED morphed in a series of five sequential morphing changes from preoperative to 3.5 years post-operative

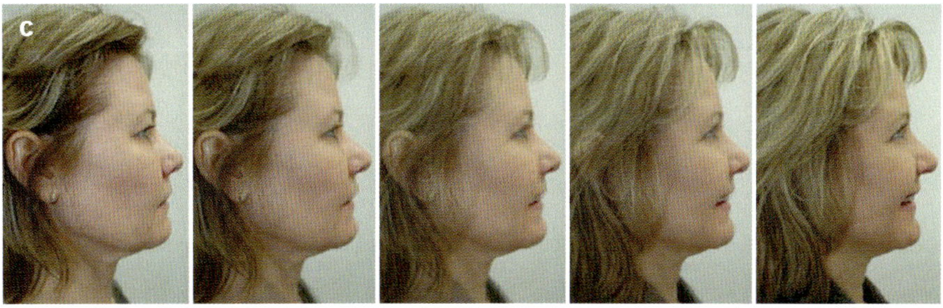

Fig. 4.42 (continued)

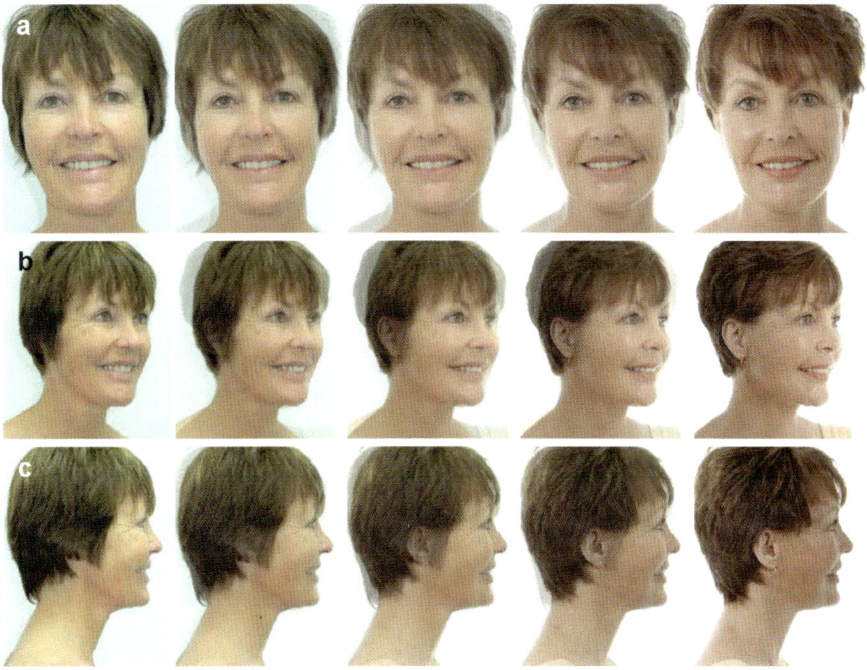

Fig. 4.43 (**a–c**) Patient PD. The face-lift of PD is morphed in a series of five sequential morphing changes from preoperative to 2.5 years post-operative

The L Ho dermal pennant flaps fixed to extra-auricular tissues have prevented malrotation of the ears and migration and distortion of the earlobe by taking the tension closure of the cervical facial flap away from the nonrigid ear and its lobe to rigid non- ear tissue. The trans-cartilaginous horizontal mattress suture provides a simple secure firm one layer closure without stitch marks (Fig. 4.40a, b). In secondary face-lift, this contour congruent procedure's dermal pennant flaps do not correct existing map rotation (Fig. 4.40c, d).

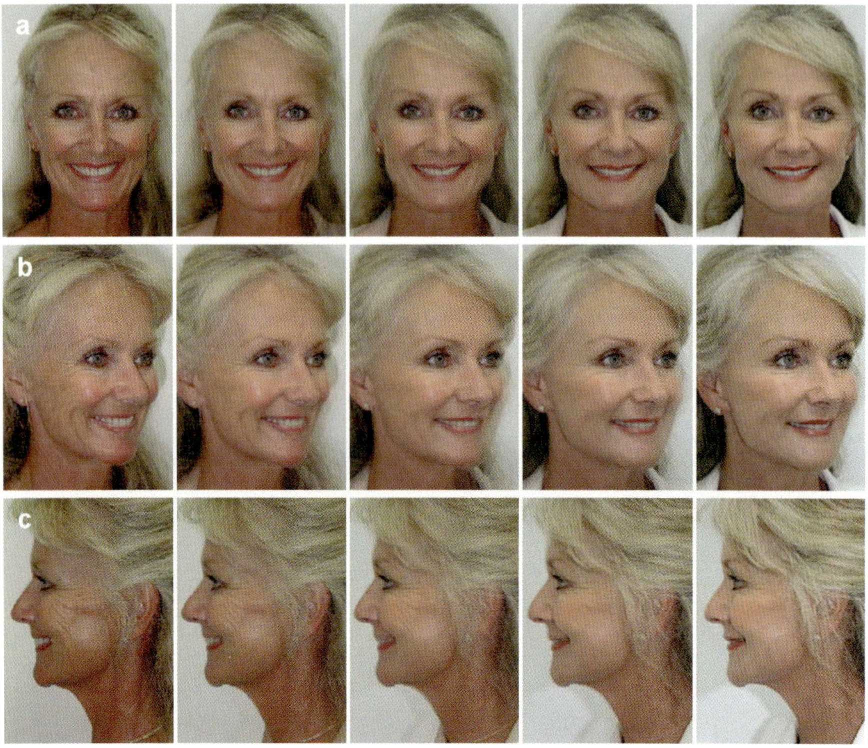

Fig. 4.44 (**a**–**c**) Patient PVC. The face-lift of PVC is morphed in a series of five morphing sequential changes from preoperative to 3 years post-operative

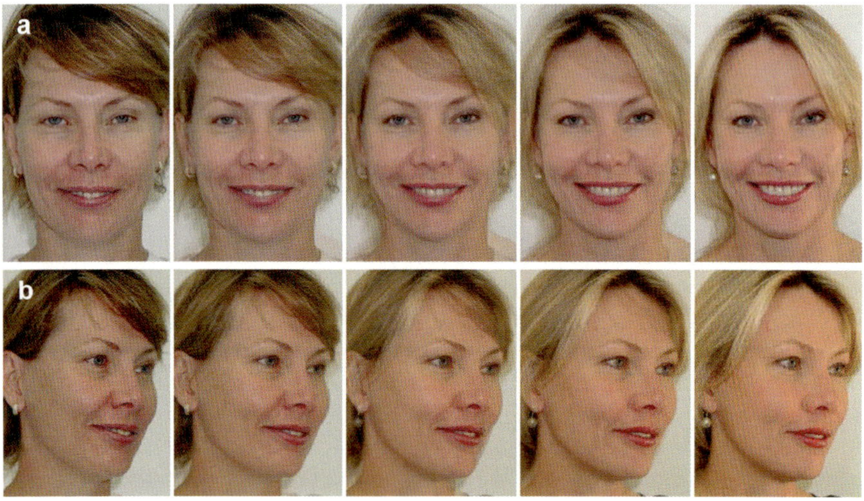

Fig. 4.45 (**a**–**c**) Patient SMH. The face-lift of SMH is morphed in changes in a series of five sequential morphing changes from preoperative to 4 years post-operative

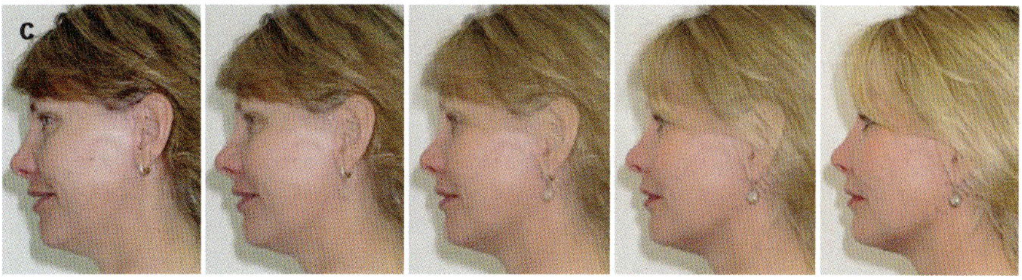

Fig. 4.45 (continued)

4.2.4 Classical Face-Lift Stigmas

The classical face-lift stigma of the popular preauricular curved skin incision extending into the temple above and posteriorly behind the ear with a largely dorsal cephalic vector across the poorly supported front/lateral plane changeover junction is the tight high-speed "wind tunnel" look. This is a four-component regional pattern stigma involving, namely, the mid- and lower face, the ear, then face/neck interphase and the upper neck. This can be grouped as the quadriga stigma pattern, the fourth "non-face" being the neck around the cervical-mental region whose stigma pattern is largely generated by local anterior platysmaplasty, mastoid tip to mastoid tip suture tightening and various lipectomies.

The mid- and lower face takes on a tight broad appearance post-operatively [3] as the trans-plane changeover junction's dorsal cephalic vector has little cephalic component for cephalic elevation of the cheek and correction of the nasolabial fold. SMAS and skin tightening traction exert tension across the front/side plane change over pilaster; this flattens its convex contour rendering a three-dimensional face into a two-dimensional planar landscape. This dorsal cephalic vector also provides little elevation in the lateral plane as well in contrast with Joseph's lateral plane face-lifts starting from 1910 which achieved a vertical skin elevation of 3.5 cm. He achieved an excellent correction of the neck and submentum. Joseph [4] delivered what Eugene Hollander's aristocratic Polish patient wanted! This is in marked contrast to Lexer [5] with his extended curvilinear preauricular incision with its dorsal cephalic vector.

Aggressive skin excision of the cervical facial skin flap with a dorsal cephalic vector delivers a ventral caudal tensioned skin flap on closure. When sewn onto the relatively mobile ear, it delivers the predictable malrotation of the ear (Fig. 4.46a) and distracted displaced elongated earlobe. The newly rediscovered unreferenced Joseph's post-tragus skin incision (1930) often adds to the list with an "open-incontinent" external meatus and a forward inclined tragus.

The strong dorsal cephalic vector from above generates an irregular fuzzy indistinct mandibular margin and angle (Fig. 4.46b) with a tented face/neck interphase [3, 6–9]. This critical region requires its own specific vector correction; its correction cannot be left over to a "rollover" effect from inadequate vector forces meant for mid- and lower face correction.

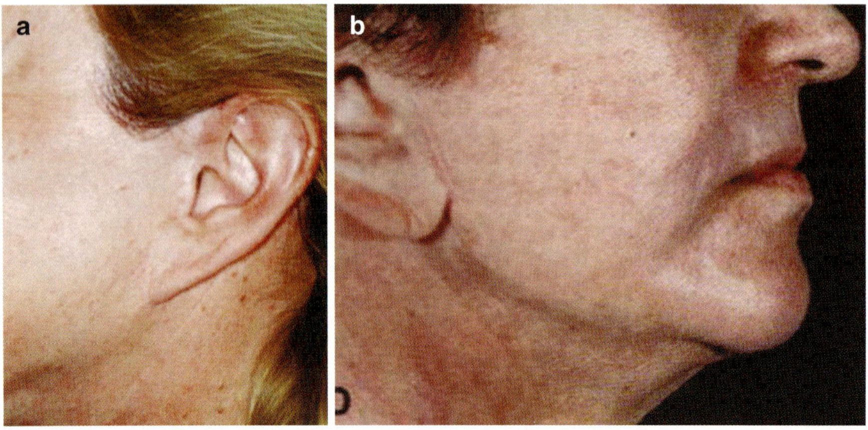

Fig. 4.46 (**a**) Ear malrotation and earlobe deformity. (**b**) Fuzzy indistinct mandibular margin and angle

Fig. 4.47 Swan neck

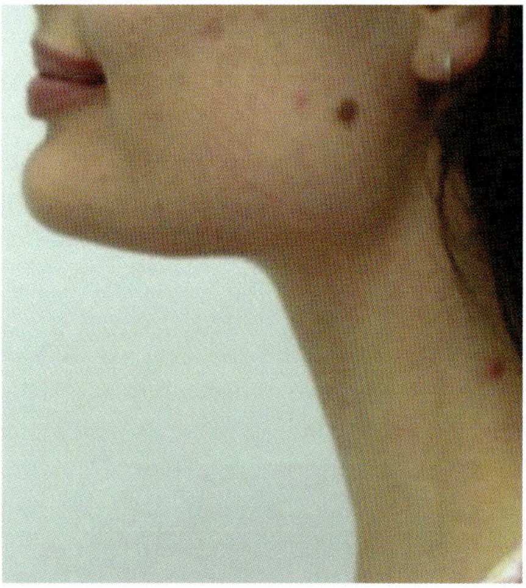

Finally, the last stigma quadriga is specific to the particular local management of the obtuse cervical-mental angle [10–12], local fat accumulation [13] and platysma band [10–14].

Each anterior platsmaplasty, mastoid tip to mastoid tip suture suspension and lipectomies inflicts its own specific tell-tale signs. Anterior platysmaplasty [10–12, 14, 15] distorts the natural smooth flow of the concave contour of the anterior upper neck. Aggressive deep para-hyoid fat lipectomy often leaves a "cavitation" at the angle in its wake. Mastoid tip to mastoid tip suspension often has a garrotting appearance; it does not produce a swan neck (Fig. 4.47).

4.2.5 Key Points

Although each contour vector congruent to enforcement loop, dermal pennant flap and trans-cartilaginous horizontal mattress suture has been designed to deliver a particular solution, they have turned out to have other benefits as well. Acting in synchrony they enhanced each other's functions, thus enhancing the overall end result. These novel features are shown below in Fig. 4.48.

Cheek Recontouring/Coning and Elevation

The cheek contour enforcement loop virtually encircles and cones the flat amorphous cheek. Elevation in the anterior plane is achieved by needling the upper limb of the loop through the zygomatic ligament and the lower limb of the loop exiting the soft tissue under the cervical facial flap after its re-entry from the buccal mucosa high up at the vertical dropped from the zygomatic eminence on the loop return. The oblique run and vector across the upper lateral plane of the face give a vertical elevation of the re-wedged and coned cheek in the front plane.

Ear Malrotation and Earlobe Distortion and Migration

These two dermal pennant flaps anchor the largely cranially vectored cervical facial flap to non-auricular tissue and prevent the said two face-lift ear stigmas. The lower

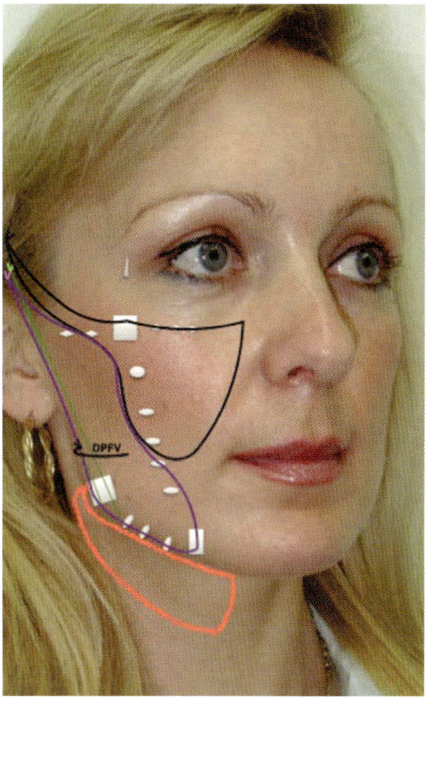

Fig. 4.48 Congruent face-lift loops and pennant flaps

dermal pennant flap is highly effective on account of its position and solely prevents earlobe distortion and untoward migration.

Crisp Smooth Mandibular Border

The rhomboid loop was designed specifically to elevate smoothly the unevenly ptosed mid- and lower face tissue and irregular bumpy mandibular margin without tension points to produce a smooth crisp smooth mandibular border (Fig. 4.49).

Its action is assisted by the cheek loop which was designed to "re-contain" and elevate the previously diffuse sagging cheek wedge. The post-operative clear sharp crisp mandibular margin is due largely to the posterior/dorsal and more importantly deep plane vectors of the lower dermal pennant flap and platysma loop; these are anchored deeply in the mastoid fascia after turning sharply inwards. Excessive tension on securing the rhomboid loop would "tent" the infra-mandibular margin and concavity causing a blurred margin. Sequence order of contribution: rhomboid loop, dermal pennant flap, platysma loop and cheek loop.

Chiselled Prominent Mandibular Angle

The rhomboid contour congruent enforcement loop positions the mandibular angle in line with the rest of the mandibular margin. Lower dermal pennant flap and platysma loop give it the sharp chiselled prominence by their deeply directed vectors. Excessive tension of narrow U-shaped and rhomboid loop will blur its margin and

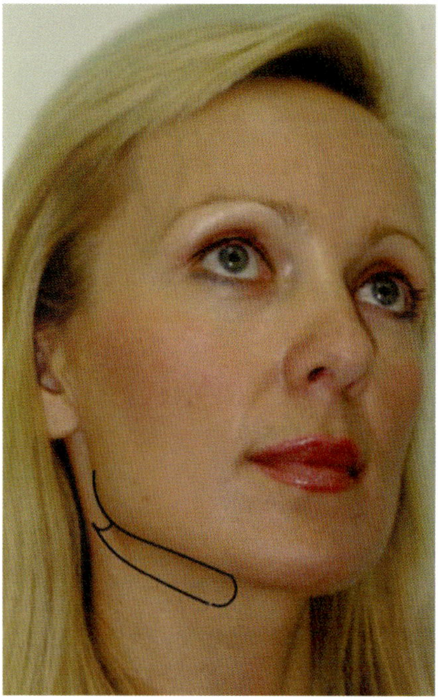

Fig. 4.49 Crisp mandibular border

definition. Sequence order of contribution is lower dermal pennant flap, congruent platysma and rhomboid loops.

Face/Neck Interphase
This delicate concave contour is restored by the crisp sharp elevation of the mandibular margin and angle, restoration of the correct length and width of the platysma and the deep thrust of the vectors of the lower dermal pennant flap and platysma loop. Sequence order of contribution is rhomboid loop, platysma loop, lower dermal pennant flap and cheek loop.

Platysma Band Correction
Rhomboid loop tightening elevation raises the platysma-auricular ligament, mandibular septa and ligament "curtain rod" to its correct youthful level (latitude), lengthening the platysma; this in turn activates its narrowing to keep volume constant. The platysma contour congruent enforcement loop narrows the platysma muscle sheet causing it to heighten further. Sequence order of contribution is rhomboid loop and platysma contour enforcement loop.

Cervical-Mental Angle
The cheek enforcement and rhomboid loops raise the lower "curtain rod" lengthening the platysma which narrows pulling the platysma band back and up and liposuction of deep para-hyoid fat pad. Sequence order of contribution of action is para-hyoid fat liposuction, rhomboid loop, platysma loop and finally the cheek loop.

Trans-cartilaginous Horizontal Matter Suture
This provides an easy firm one layer secure skin closure without leaving suture marks on easily visible part of the face.

4.2.6 Ageing Pathology Components

Ageing fat compartment de-voluming and ligament septa attenuation set in motion ptotic gravitation migration of fat compartments along predetermined channels of the weakened system of support generating the well-recognised stigma pattern. Often these two processes do not proceed concurrently at the same pace. When skin laxity is slight or moderate, rejuvenation may be achieved by accurate precise correction of individual fat compartment soft tissue volume deficit [16]. This activates a gravitational fat compartment remigration to a youthful latitude and longitude along the re-energised existing network of ligaments and septa by precise "reflation" of the appropriate individual fat compartments. This achieves what the congruent contour enforce loop system has been designed to achieve where ptosis is a prominent component of the pathology; it is only applicable where there is little redundant skin. This procedure is rejuvenative facial lipomorphoplasty [16]. The mid- and lower face's unique support structure with its soft tissue and fat secured into

compartments has been utilised in the above technique for rejuvenation of the aged face when there is little skin excess. It has also been utilised to optimise the appearance of the face in facial optimisation [17]**.**

The feasibility and consistent reproducibility of the quality obtained from this technical procedure suggest that the described large compartments are themselves built up of little compartment blocks which allow for accurate reconstruction and realignment of pilasters to restore the position, size, incline and robust crispness and the youthful change in appearance of the face. Further investigation will be required to confirm this. Advantage of this suggested structure has been utilised with facial optimisation [17].

4.3 Rejuvenative Facial Lipomorphoplasty

The face is a three-dimensional anatomical structure. Its front and two side planes have been described earlier in Chap. 2. The major front and side planes have a changeover junction which is 80° and is secured by the oblique line of zygomatic and masseter ligaments and septa. Changeover junctions of major planes are primary pilasters (black); changeover junctions of minor or sub-planes and facial features (eyebrow) are secondary pilasters (red). These are recapitulated in Fig. 4.50. Pilasters are seen visually and in photographs as highlight borders or margins [16–21].

Ageing drives changes in facial planes and sub-planes, primary and secondary pilasters from age de-voluming of progressive fat and soft tissue atrophy, ligament/septa attenuation and lengthening and skin laxity. The facial pilasters [16] become progressively less robust and undergo changes in position, incline, size, shape,

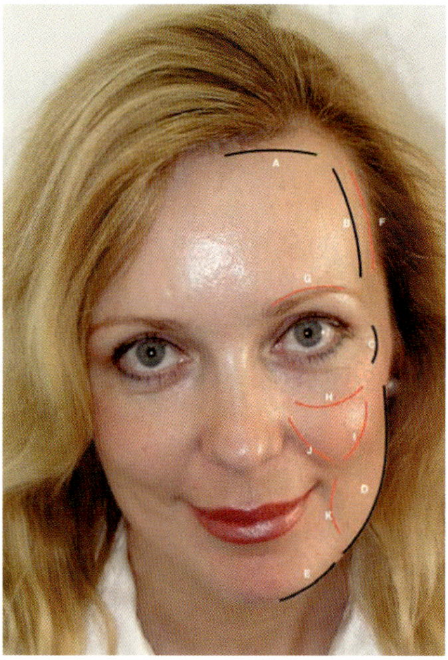

Fig. 4.50 Age pilasters. Changes drive plane changes which generate the age stigmas (Video 4.6)

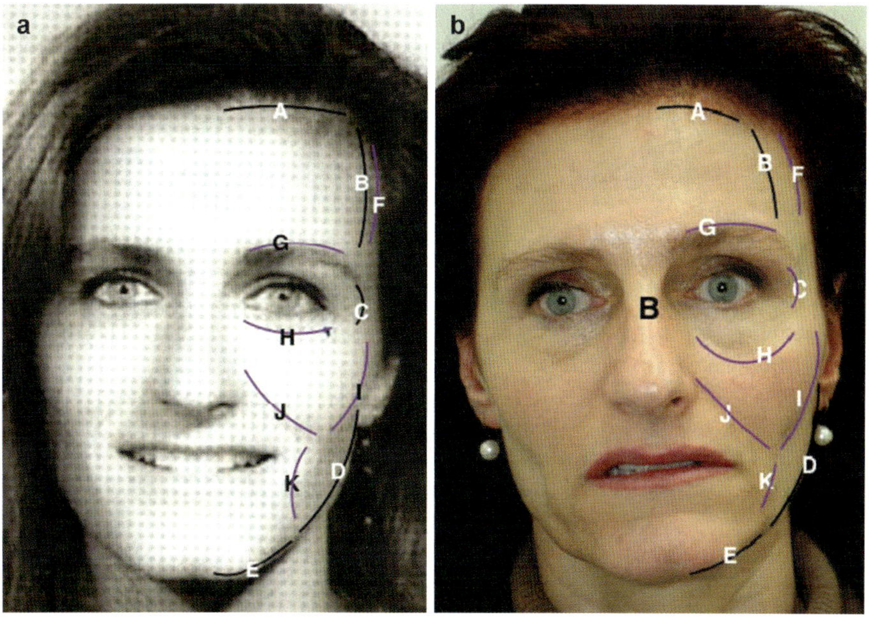

Fig. 4.51 (**a**) Template with pilasters (Video 4.7) (**b**) Current pilasters (Video 4.8)

configuration and robustness; these in turn drive changes of the planes and sub-planes which generate the stigma of the ageing face, expression and smile; these are functions of positioned muscle excursion and not viscoelastic changes. However these two processes of sagging and de-voluming do not proceed synchronously. Some aged faces exhibit significant sagging, but a significant percentage suffers from gaunt ageing with little soft tissue and skin sagging. This category does not fare well from face-lifting but benefits greatly from restoration of structural volume deficit with autogenous fat transplant [16]. Figure 4.51a, b demonstrates gaunt ageing changes from age 20 to 47.

Management of these patients by adequate restoration of structural volume deficit with autogenous fat micro grafts inflates the fat compartments. This restores fullness and firmness and tightens the slack ligaments which in turn restructure the pilasters, planes and sub-planes to their more youthful shape, robustness and position; this is the technique of choice.

4.3.1 Operative Technique

4.3.1.1 Fat Micro Graft Harvesting and Preparation

The procedure is performed under sedation and local anaesthetic nerve blocks with an anaesthetist in attendance. Approximately 250 ml of fat micro grafts is harvested with a hub cannula and 60 ml syringe. Donor sites are the regions where fat hypertrophies in middle and old age and around regions rich in vascular supply, i.e. the upper inner thighs and abdomen around the perforator vessels. These micro grafts are transferred to 10 ml Luer-Lock syringes and stood in a rack for 1 h to allow sedimentation separation. During this time completion pump liposuction is performed to smooth the donor sites' contour. The serum at the bottom and the oil floating at the top are removed by gentle syringe aspiration. The stab incisions are closed, donor sites dressed and the patient is next positioned for structural volume restoration.

4.3.1.2 Structural Volume Restoration and Pilaster Reconstruction

The previously well-scrutinised current and old photos are restudied, and a suitable template and current photos in five views both smiling and static are displayed on the operating room wall for reference during the procedure. Multiple small access stab incisions are made for precise accurate placement of the fat micro grafts on each side for structural volume deficit restoration and accurate precise pilaster reconstruction and realignment. A fine three-hole bullet-headed cannula mounted on a 10 ml small volume (0.2 ml) delivery injection gun is used for precise placement of the micro grafts. These are delivered in multiple layers in a grid pattern to build up each aesthetic unit. Bilateral aesthetic units are built up on both sides symmetrically before moving to the next unit till completion of face volume restoration bilaterally. Precise adequate correction of the structural volume deficit of each facial feature inflates each fat compartment, elevating the dermal insertion points of the ligaments and septa to the latitude of their origin reorientating the relevant pilasters to a more youthful position and shape as indicated in the template photograph on the wall. This pilaster reconstruction generates secondary changes to the facial planes and sub-planes which in turn drive the youthful changes in the appearance of the face. As there is no complete vascularisation and taking of the fat micro grafts, overcorrection is performed to compensate for this. The face is 15% and lips 30% overcorrected. The much greater overcorrection of the lips is due to its frequent movements in the post-operative recovery period. Excess fat is stored in tissue culture medium at 4 °C in the fridge. This is used at 4 weeks for top-up or touch-up of any asymmetries and inadequacies.

The face and neck are thoroughly cleansed and dried. The stab incisions are steristriped and an appropriate head dressing is applied. The patient is discharged later in the day when fit or may stay overnight. Steristrips and dressing are removed 10 days post-operatively. Touch-up and top-up are performed at 4 weeks if required.

4.3.2 Case Studies

The following five case examples illustrate the average result of a sizeable number of patients who have undergone the described procedure. **The goal of rejuvenative facial lipomorphoplasty is to produce a full, youthful, firm and youthfully repositioned face structure with clean-cut, well-defined reconstructed pilasters, planes and sub-planes. Lax ptotic cheeks, indistinct front/lateral plane changeover junctions, ptosed eyebrows, hollow temples and eyes and weak irregular mandibular margin and angles should be restored and refined.** The following case examples illustrate a number of patients who have undergone the described procedure. A critical look at the after images will allow the reader to pick up shortfalls in the operative technique performed by the senior surgeon author.

An optimum long-lasting result requires correct choice of donor site, atraumatic harvesting and handling of the fat micro grafts and accurate atraumatic

placement of micro grafts to ensure early vascularisation. This requires good clinical judgement and experience (Figs. 4.52, 4.53, 4.54, 4.55, 4.56, 4.57, 4.58, 4.59, 4.60 and 4.61).

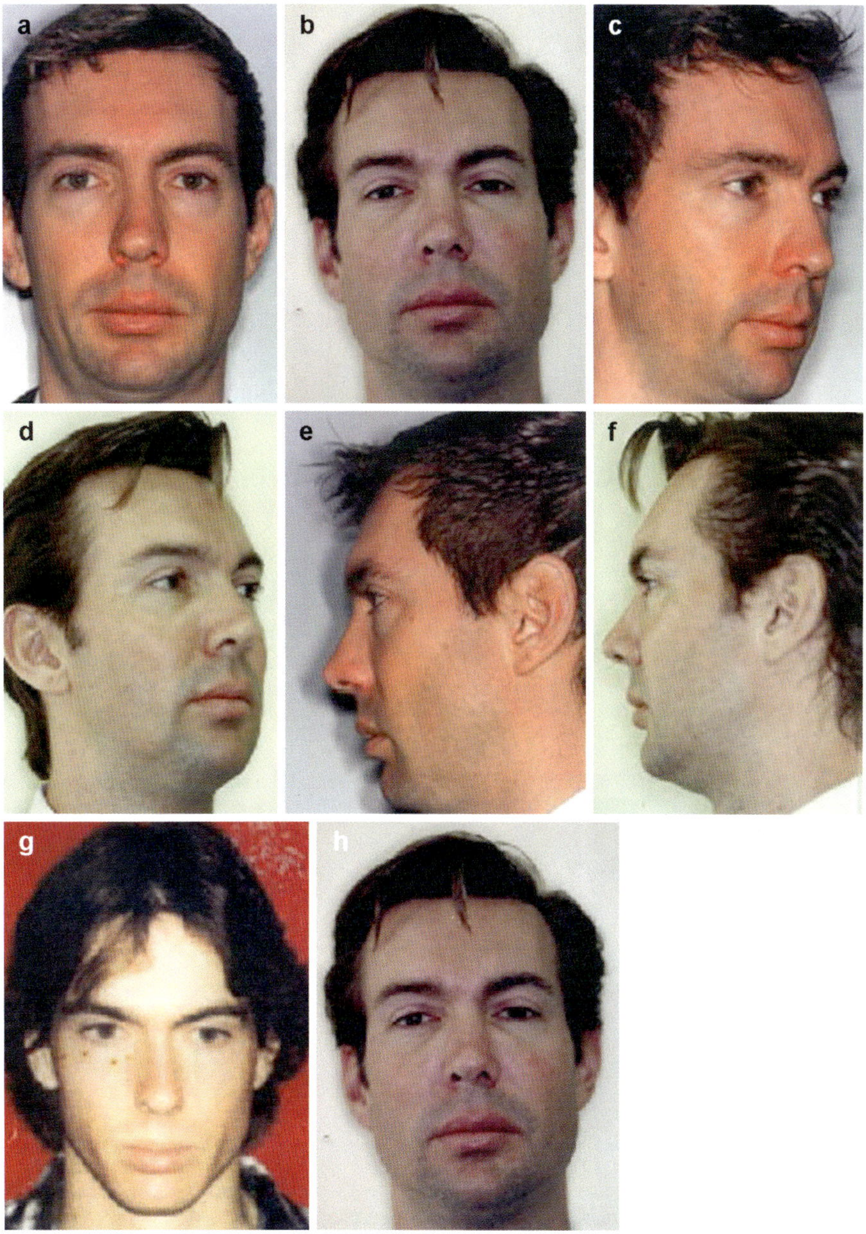

Fig. 4.52 Patient JN (first patient) aged 34. Presented in 1997; said "I want a face-lift but not a face-lift"; showed photo (**g**) in bottom left at age 18. (**a**, **c**, **e**) Before. (**b**, **d**, **f**, **h**) Post-operative follow-up photos in 2000 aged 37 years. Volume replacement: 120 ml at primary procedure; 24 ml at touch-up at 4 weeks

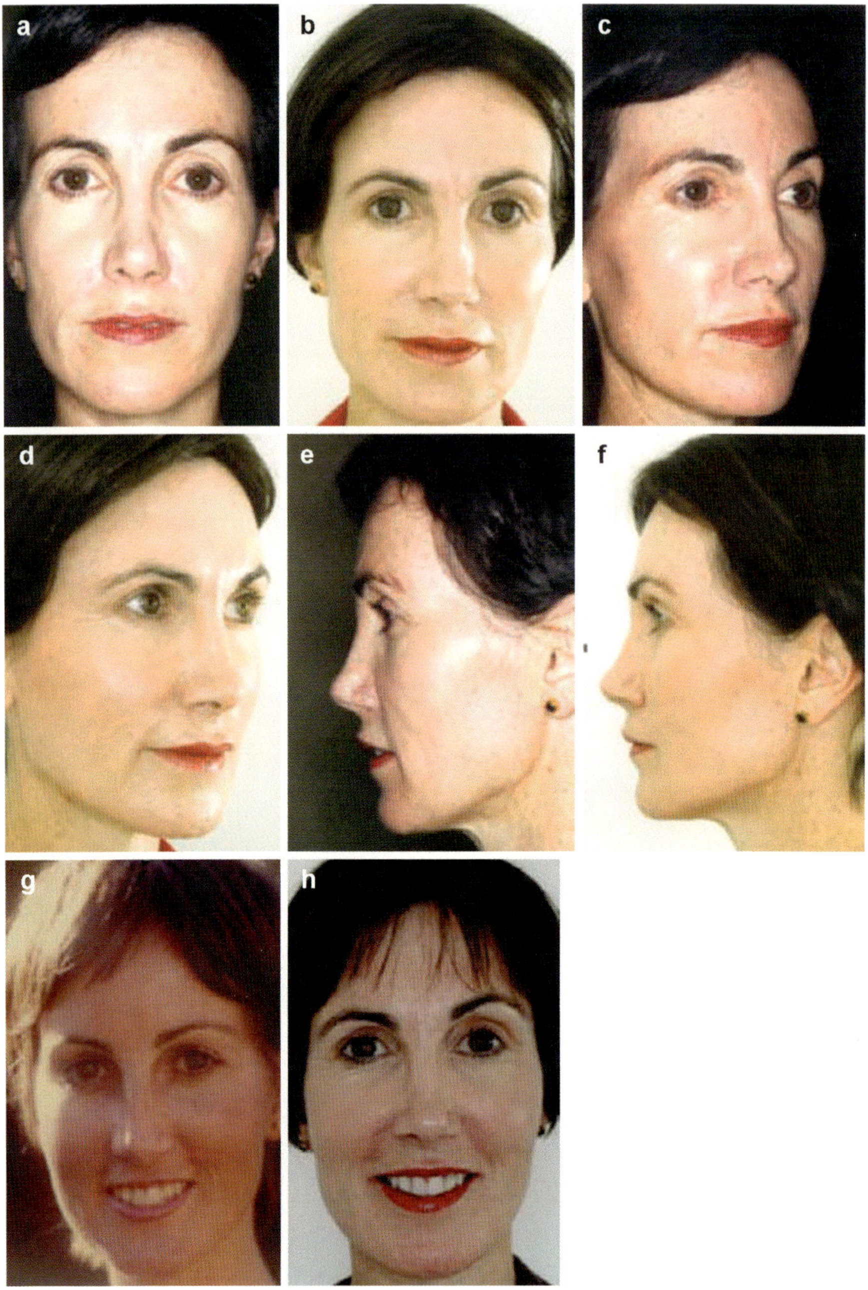

Fig. 4.53 Patient LH Template 18 years. (**a**, **c**, **e**) Age 49 years with gaunt ageing. (**b**, **d**, **f**, **h**) 51 years. (**g**) 18 years. Volume replacement: 85 ml of fat used (*Adapted from Ho* [16])

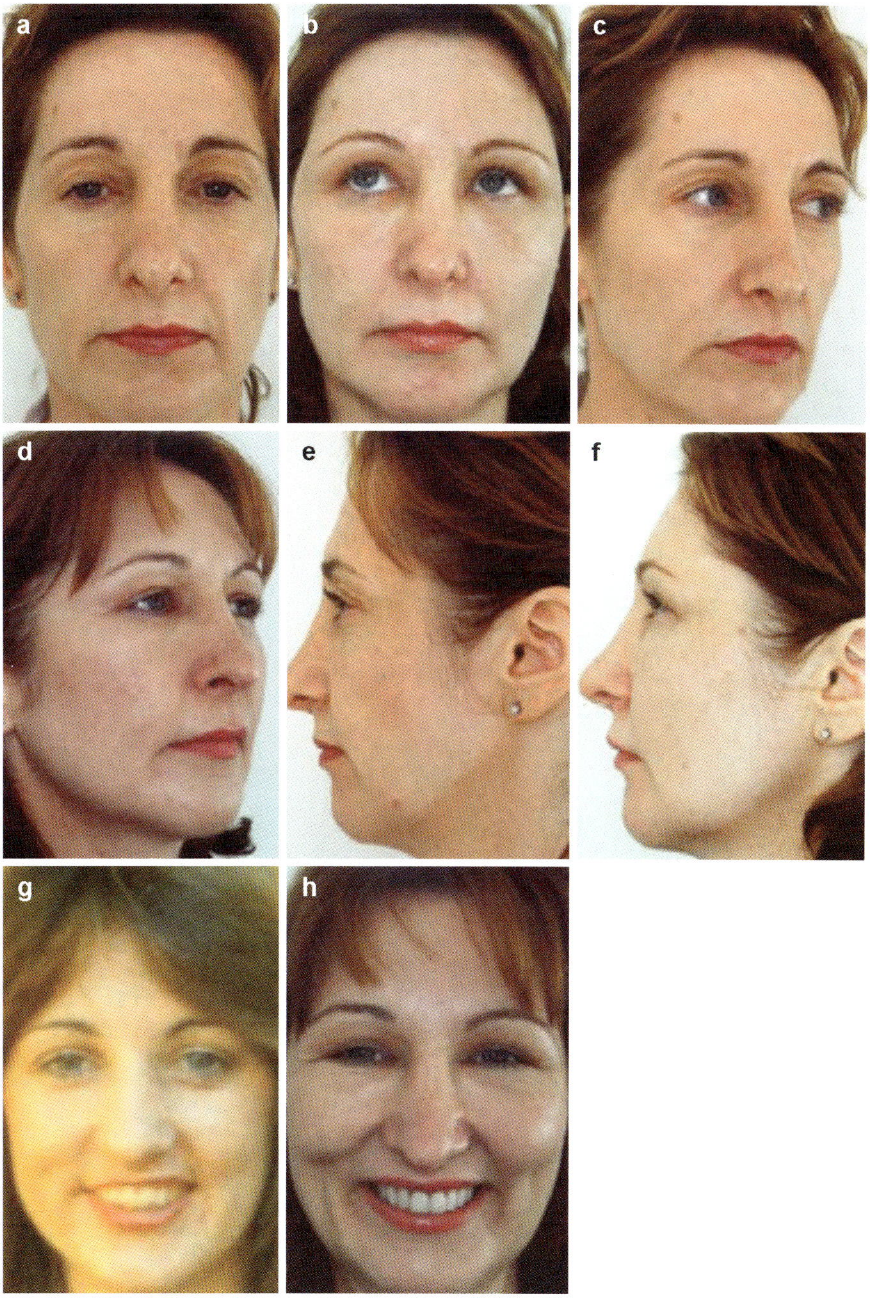

Fig. 4.54 Patient PW. (**g**) aged 18.(**a**, **c**, **e**) 41 years, (**b**, **d**, **f**, **h**) 43 years. Marked fat atrophy. Volume replacement 190 ml fat (*Adapted from Ho* [16])

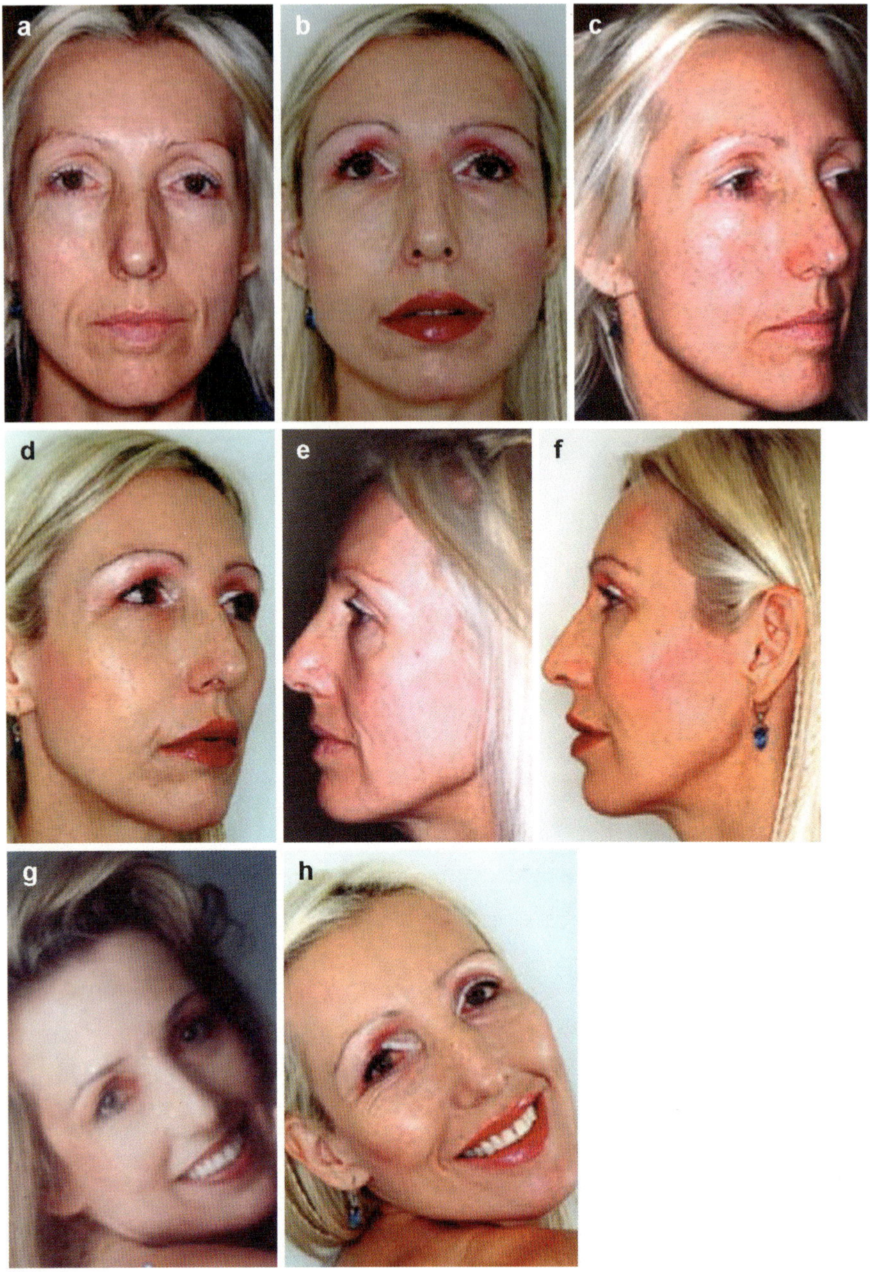

Fig. 4.55 Patient HD (**g**) age 21 years. (**a**, **c**, **e**) 47 years. (**b**, **d**, **f**, **h**) 51 years. Volume replacement 175 ml

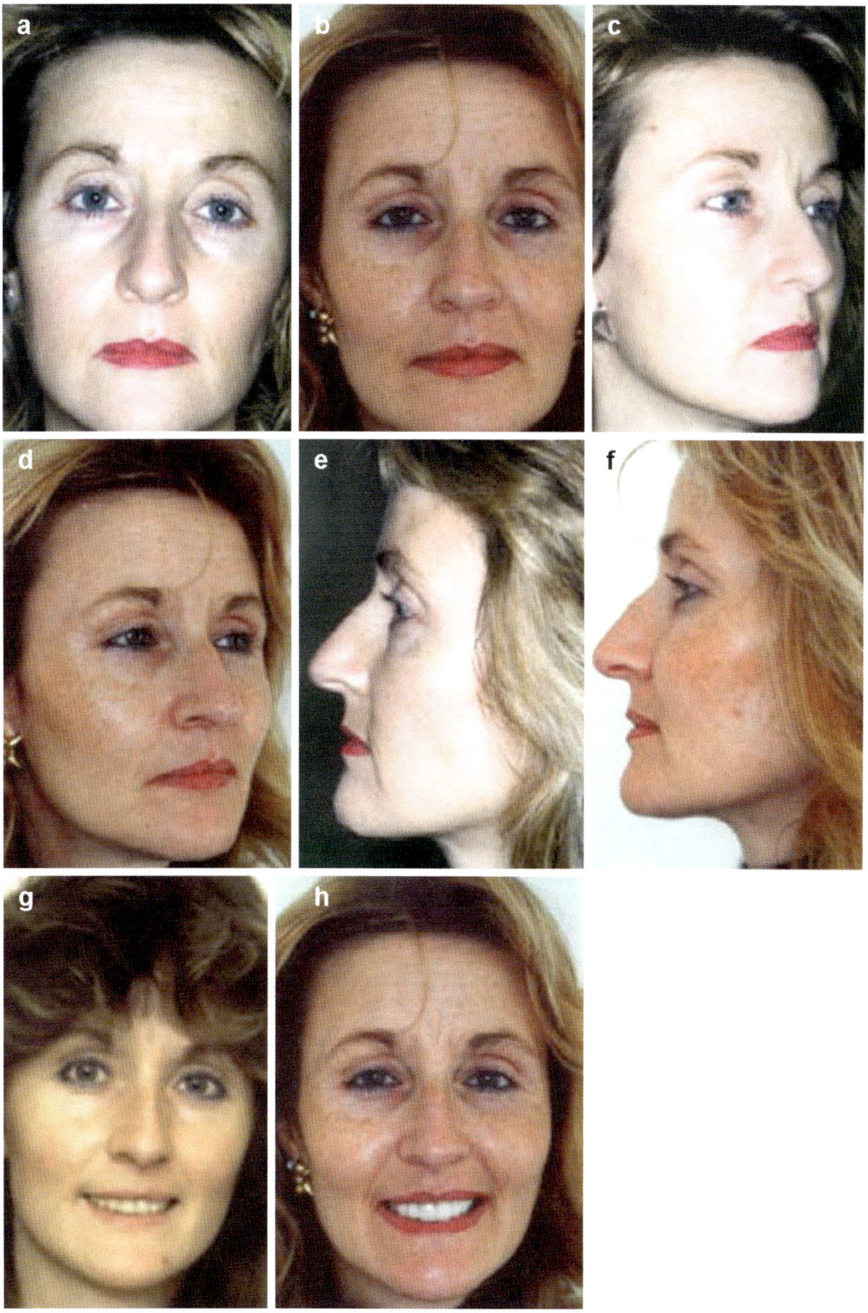

Fig. 4.56 Patient PA (**g**) age 19 years, (**a**, **c**, **e**) Before 43 years, (**b**, **d**, **f**, **h**) 48 years. Volume replacement 165 ml

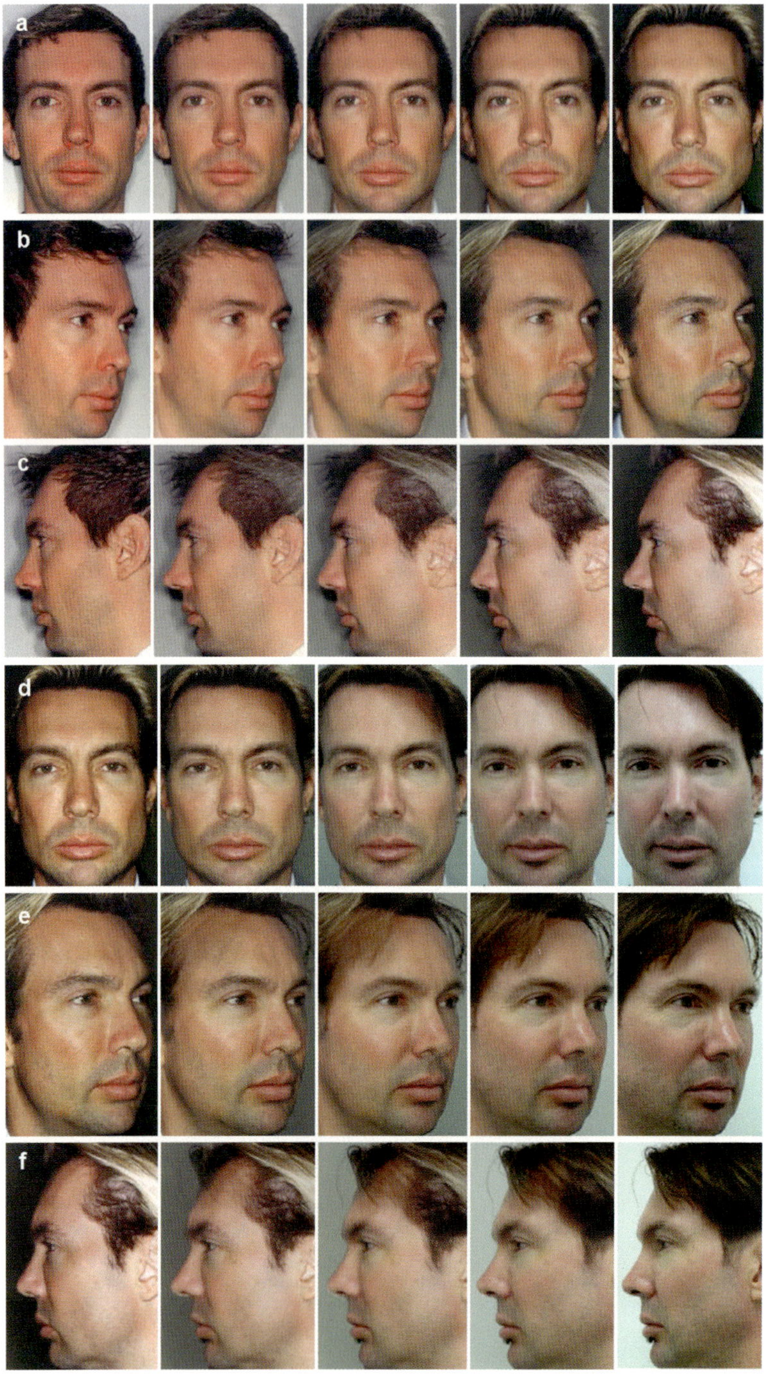

Fig. 4.57 (**a–c**) Rejuvenative facial lipomorphoplasty sequential morphing changes from presentation to follow-up in three views. Patient JN presented in 1997 age 34. Follow-up right 2005 age 41 years (and finally at age 47 years in next series). (**d–f**) Patient JN further progressive facial changes from 41 to 47 years in three views driven by fat de-voluming generating secondary changes of pilasters and facial planes and sub-planes

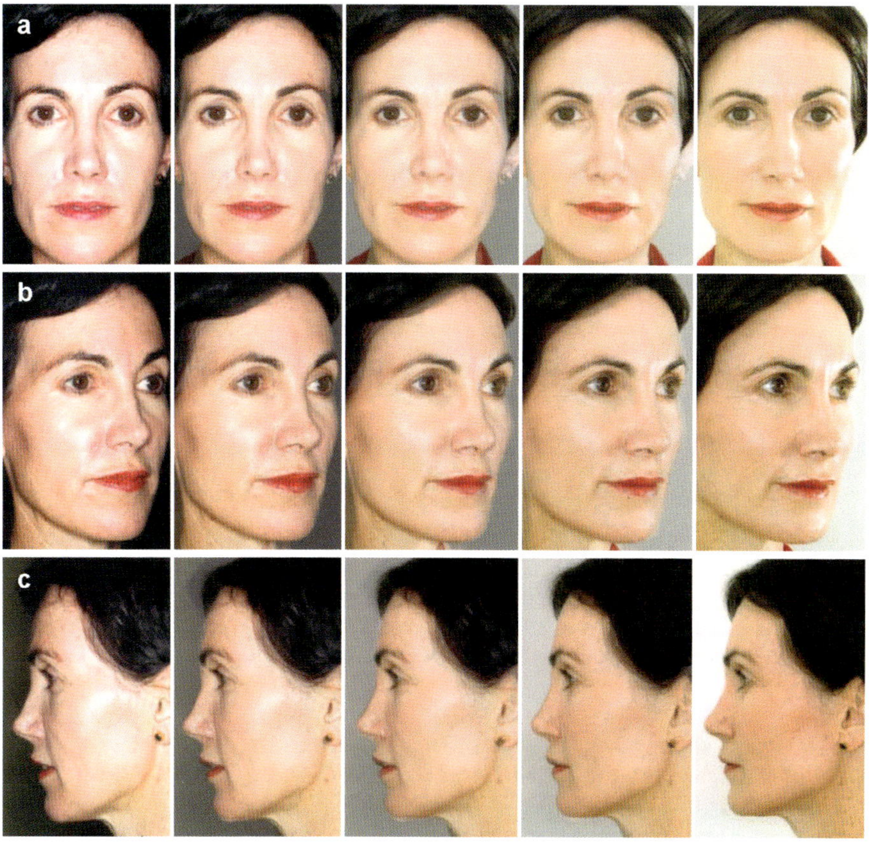

Fig. 4.58 (**a–c**) Patient LH. Sequential morphing changes from presentation at age 47 to follow up at age 49 in three views

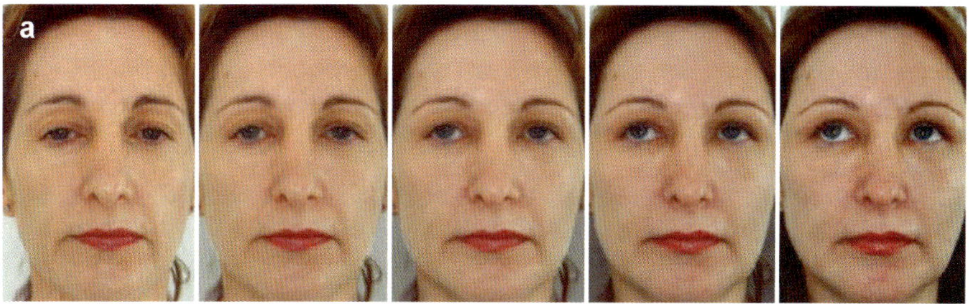

Fig. 4.59 (**a–c**) Patient PW. Sequential morphing changes from presentation at age 41 to follow up at age 43 in three views

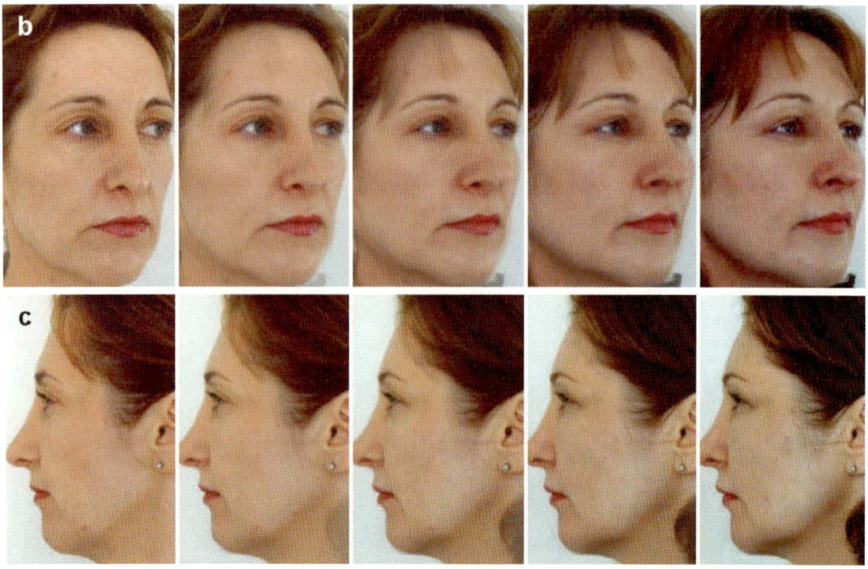

Fig. 4.59 (continued)

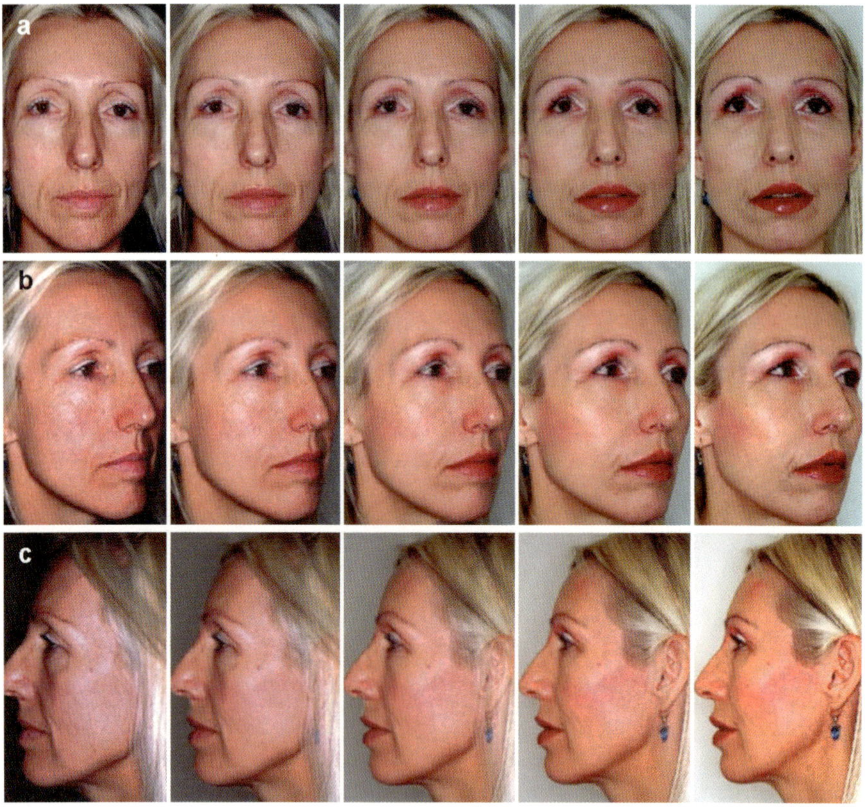

Fig. 4.60 (**a–c**) Patient HD. Sequential morphing changes from presentation at age 47 to follow up at 51 in three views

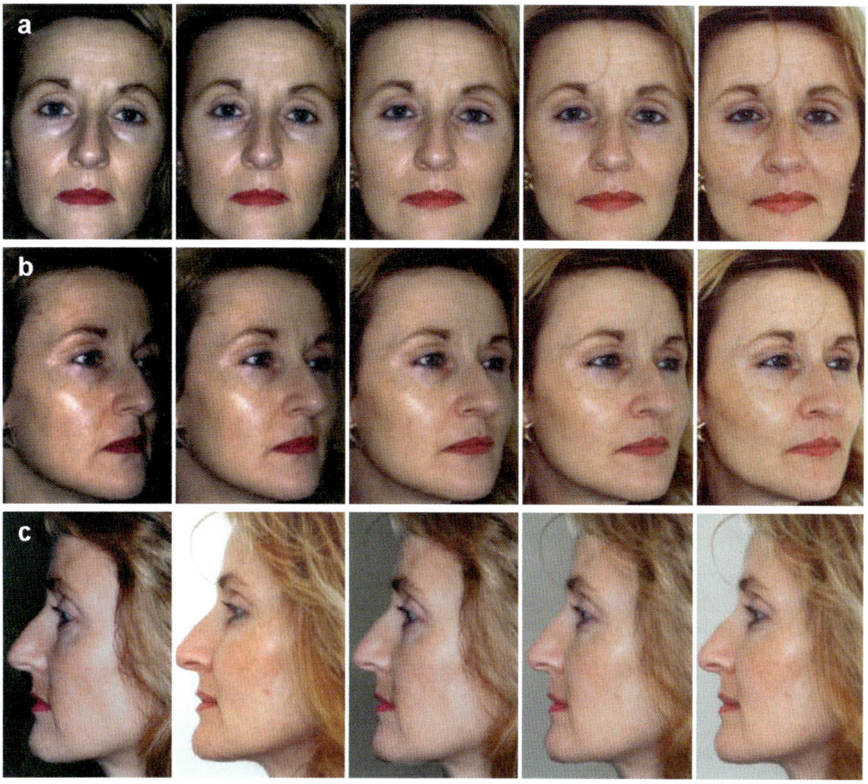

Fig. 4.61 (**a–c**) Patient PA Sequential morphing changes from presentation at age 43 to follow up at age 48 in three views

4.3.3 Key Points

Donor (Fat) Site Choice

Optimum sites—regions which undergo hypertrophy with ageing, i.e. lower abdomen, hips and upper thighs.

Areas near vascular structures are rich in stroma cells, adipoblasts and stem cells.

Transplanted autogenous cells retain growth behaviour of region of origin.

Recipient bed cells continue to atrophy.

Good volume maintenance with progressive ageing achieved with optimal donor/recipient ratio.

Atraumatic Harvesting and Handling of Grafts

Syringe aspiration harvesting.

Sedimentation for separation of fractions.

Use of cell culture medium for storage at 4 °C.

Microinjection of Fat Micro Grafts

Injection gun mounted syringe—2 ml syringe for eyelids and eyebrow.

Multihole bullet nose cannula.

Patient template photo on wall guide to adequacy of volume correction.
Multilevel layering injection of each aesthetic unit.
Adequate aesthetic re-voluming each aesthetic to reconstruct relevant pilaster.

Prophylaxis Against Intravascular Injection Misadventure
Digital compression of adjacent vascular bundles at injection.
Inject on withdrawal of syringe.
Do not inject deep to orbital septum.

Injection Volume Judgement
Entirely visual—aesthetic unit/feature full and firm; pilaster alignment.
Sunken upper eyelids require 2–3 ml (in subcutaneous plane).
85% overcorrection.
At finish face should match template photo on wall.

Sequential Injection Volume Restoration
Re-volume paired aesthetic units of the face sequentially.
Start with cheeks (runs around plane change over junction) and lower eyelids.
Then orbito-temporo-zygomatic region, frontal temporal pilaster region, temporal fossa, forehead and then down to lower face.

How Long Does It Last? (JN Series: Fig. 4.62a–e)
The first patient treated by this technique (JN) demonstrates in the 2-year postoperative photos (and subsequent photos) volume correction was inadequate in the temple and lateral forehead regions but adequate in the mid- and lower face. Over the following 11 years, this difference is maintained. Progressing over the years with recipient bed face fat atrophy and ligament/septa attenuation and lengthening, sagging develops with realignment of pilasters and consequent facial appearance. Adequately re-volumed features were fairly well maintained at 13 years post-procedure but suffer from age sagging.

The university entrance photo taken at the age of 18 years shows some gauntness. The ageing series after rejuvenative facial lipomorphoplasty would suggest more facial fat padding a couple of years earlier at age 16. Unfortunately, the patient did not have any relevant photos taken 2 or 3 years earlier. The temples are hollow and sunken at 47, a testimony to inadequate volume correction here. The cheek, double chin and jowls remain well corrected, and the mandibular margin and angles are distinct, clean-cut and crisp.

How Useful Is the Template Photograph?
Patients would like to look more youthful and younger but not different. As the result is controlled by the visual appearance of the face during the operative procedure, it is important to ascertain from the patient what he or she would look like timeframe wise in their life. There is often a period look in their facial appearance which look back fondly to.

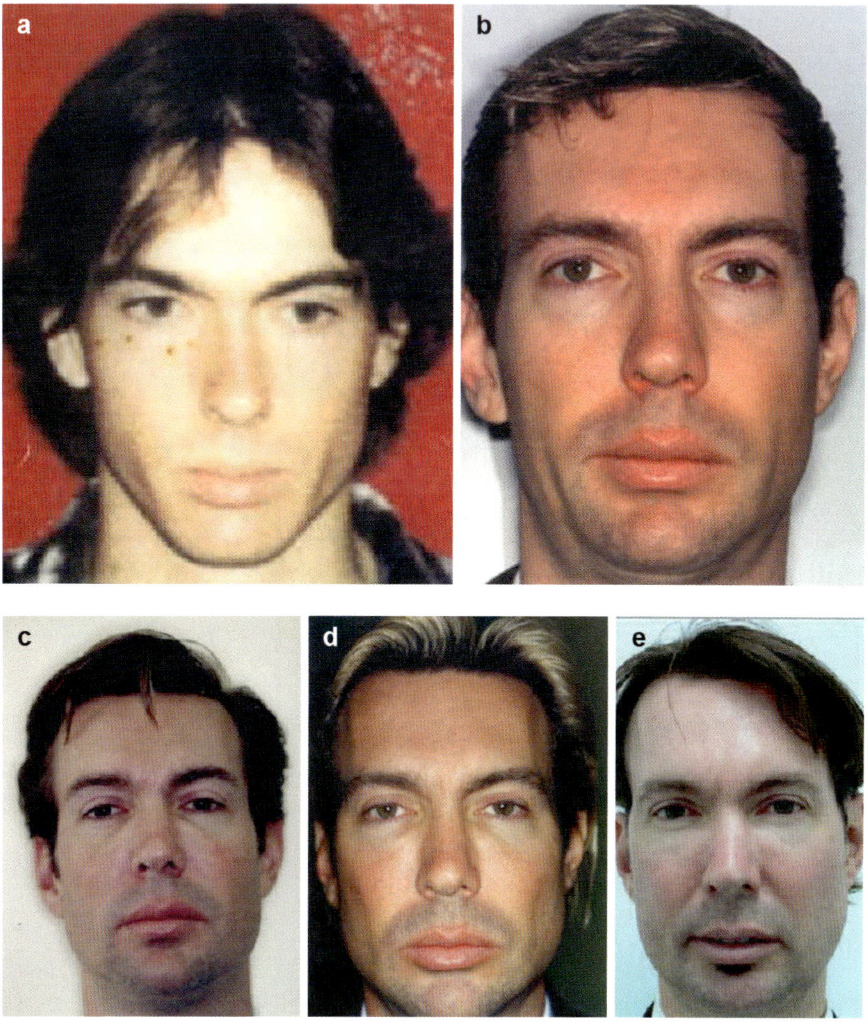

Fig. 4.62 (**a**) Template aged 18. (**b**) Presentation at age 34. (**c–e**) Progressive changes at follow-up in 2000 at age 37, 2005 at age 41 and 2011 at age 47

PW Series (Fig. 4.63a–e)

PW brought along old shown in Fig. 4.63b, c; chose Fig. 4.63b as template. It was all she had at home of an early photo and volunteered that her face had shrunk considerably over the years. Three weeks after the procedure, it was noticed that the face was overcorrected (Fig. 4.63e) in relation to the template at age 26. When asked if she had any earlier photos, 3 months later, she brought in a small photo taken at age 18 years from her mother's home in New South Wales 500 miles away. It would appear that injection of fat micro grafts to fully fill the facial skin envelope took it to the maximum volume in the patient's life; in this case it was age 18 years.

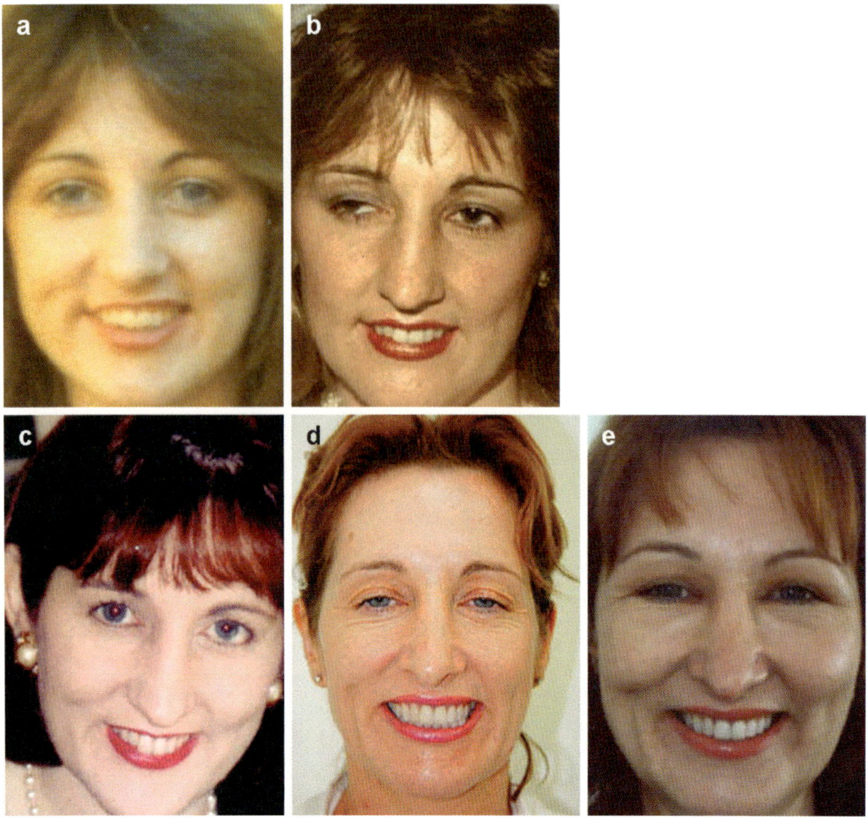

Fig. 4.63 (**a**) Age 18 (**b**) Age 26 (**c**) Age 32 (**d**) Age 41 (**e**) Age 43. Patient PW presented at age 41 years with two old photos as templates aged 26 and 32. Chosen template was (**b**) aged 26. Result (**e**) did not match (**b**) but (**a**), aged 18 which she retrieved 3 months after the procedure

4.4 Facial Optimisation

Precisely targeted injection of the appropriate volume of fat micro grafts is used to alter existing unaesthetic facial pilaster size, position and incline to drive changes in the size, shape and relative positions of the facial planes and sub-planes to produce a more aesthetic face shape and appearance.

The mid- and lower face's unique support structure with its soft tissue and fat secured into compartments reflects the borders of the facial planes and sub-planes. In the upper face, this compartmentation is repeated; instead of ligaments and septa, the separation is effected by (fibrous) adhesions of deep dermis to the underlying periosteum. These described compartments appear to be built of little subunit blocks. This allows for aesthetic recruitment of adjacent compartment subunits to effect a reconstructive change in size, shape, position and incline of relevant pilasters which in turn drives aesthetic changes in the size, shape and orientation of the planes and

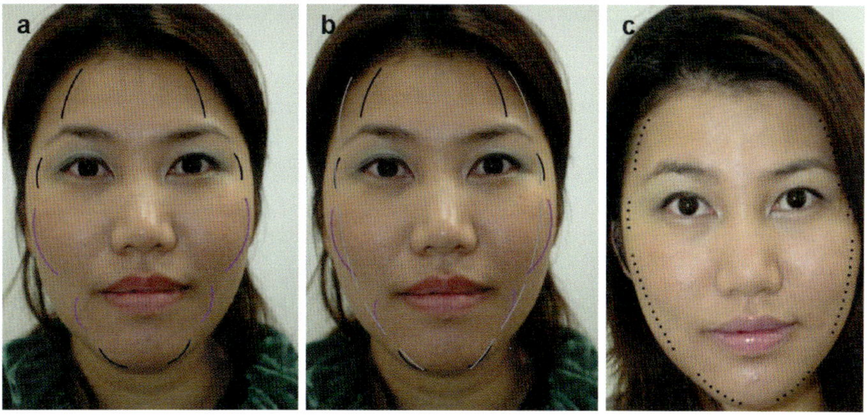

Fig. 4.64 (**a**) Pilasters: major in black minor on lilac (**b**) Proposed pilasters in grey (Video 4.9) (**c**) New oval face

sub-planes into a more congruent aesthetic integration of these sub-planes and planes. The eye does not see details but only margin or border highlights (pilasters) of planes and sub-planes. Highlights reinforce their impression in the visual cortex by the phenomenon of lateral inhibition of adjacent un-bright areas [19–21].

4.4.1 Methods and Operative Technique

At consultation images of the face (smiling and at rest) are taken in front, left and right oblique and lateral views. These are viewed with the patient. Existing pilasters are marked out on the images (Fig. 4.64a); these pilasters are highlight margins of planes and sub-planes.

The patient's desired appearance is ascertained; the proposed new pilasters are marked out on the image on the Keynote app (originally on the photo) in grey as shown in this case in Fig. 4.64b.

Precise construction of the proposed new pilasters should produce the following planned desired result shown in Fig. 4.64c as the bilateral rows of reconstructed pilaster highlights would have been realigned congruently [16, 17]. *Fat micro graft harvesting and preparation* are similar that for rejuvenative lipomorphoplasty [16].

Facial Optimisation: Pilaster Reconstruction

The paper printouts of the images with existing and proposed new pilaster lines in the front, oblique and side views are placed on a convenient operating room wall for easy reference during the procedure. Small access stab incisions are made for precise accurate placement of the fat micro grafts on each side of the face for reconstruction/relocation of new pilaster lines. The technique is similar to that described previously for rejuvenative lipomorphoplasty [16]. Reconstruction commences from the forehead and moves caudally after completing aesthetic units of both sides. The proposed new frontal temporal pilaster is built up by serial delivery of small volumes of fat micro grafts with the injection gun along the proposed pilaster line. When the new pilaster ridge is finished, the contour deficiency between this ridge and existing pilaster is filled in to smooth. Following this, the other side of the new pilaster ridge is microinjected to smooth off the contour. The opposite new frontal temporal pilaster ridge is similarly constructed and smoothed on both sides. The existing frontal vertex pilaster is reinforced and tensioned. New pilaster construction proceeds caudally on each side in sequence from orbital-temporal-zygomatic pilaster, lateral cheek pilaster, oral-masseteric pilaster and finally the mental pilaster. Precise aesthetic reconstruction of new pilasters to a more congruent integrated pleasing architectural frame is performed. This pilaster reconstruction generates secondary changes to the facial planes and sub-planes which in turn drives the aesthetic changes in the appearance of the face. As full vascularisation and taking of the injected fat micro grafts are not guaranteed, 15% overcorrection is performed. Excess fat is stored in tissue culture medium at 4 °C in the fridge; this is used at 4 weeks for touch-up of any shortfalls at the primary procedure.

The face and neck are thoroughly cleansed and dried. The stab incisions are steristriped and an appropriate head dressing is applied. The patient is discharged later in the day when fit or may stay overnight. Steristrips and dressing are removed 10 days post-operatively. Touch-up is performed at 4 weeks if required.

4.4.2 Case Studies

Four case examples illustrate the average result of a small series of patients who have undergone the described procedure. A critical look at the before/after images will allow the reader to pick up shortfalls in the operative technique performed by the senior surgeon author (Figs. 4.65, 4.66, 4.67, 4.68, 4.69, 4.70, 4.71 and 4.72).

4.4.3 Key Points

Cheek (Fig. 4.73a, b)
Oblique angulated (80°) biplane (front largely and side) long tapering wedge feature across the midface.

Straddles five fat compartments—medial and middle cheek, inferior orbital, lateral orbital and lateral temporal—cheek compartments.

Recruits only small parts of four compartments into its structure.

Transgresses across zygomatic ligament, septa and inferior temporal septum without break in continuity of form.

Early break in wedge integrity/continuity in front plane by buccal maxillary septa generated oblique sulcus running from medial canthus.

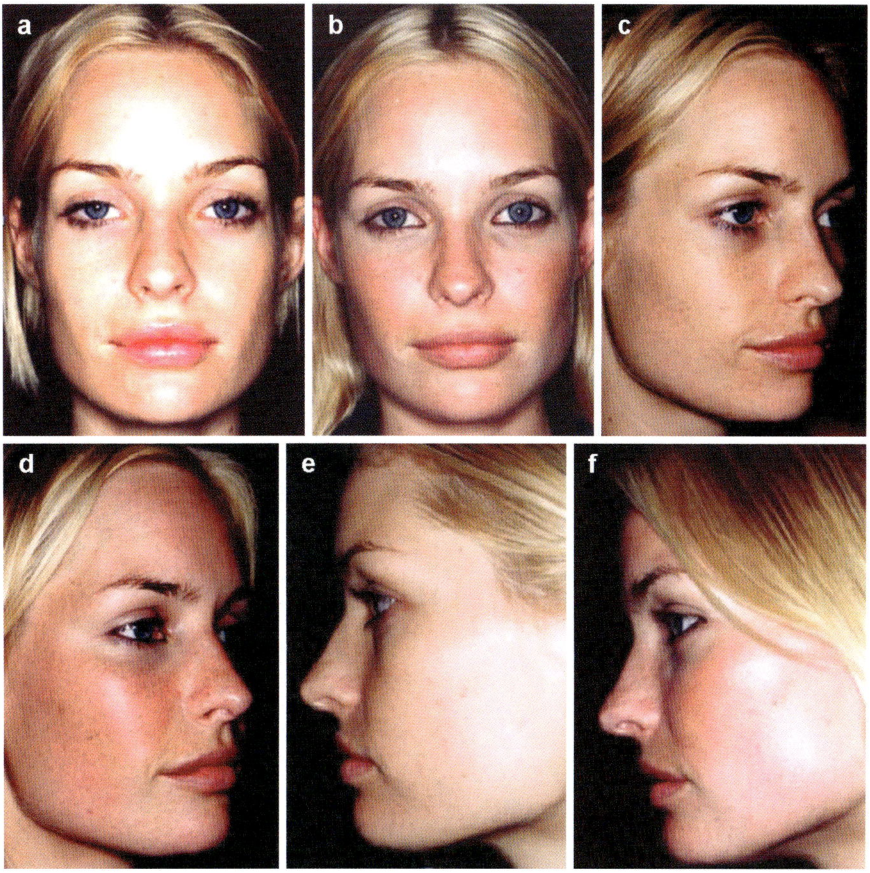

Fig. 4.65 Patient LJ presented in 1999 at age 23 years asking to be made to look better and fresh. (**a**, **c**, **e**) Before. (**b**, **d**, **f**) Post-operative follow-up photos right in 2001 aged 25 years. Volume used for facial optimisation (first patient) was 85 ml

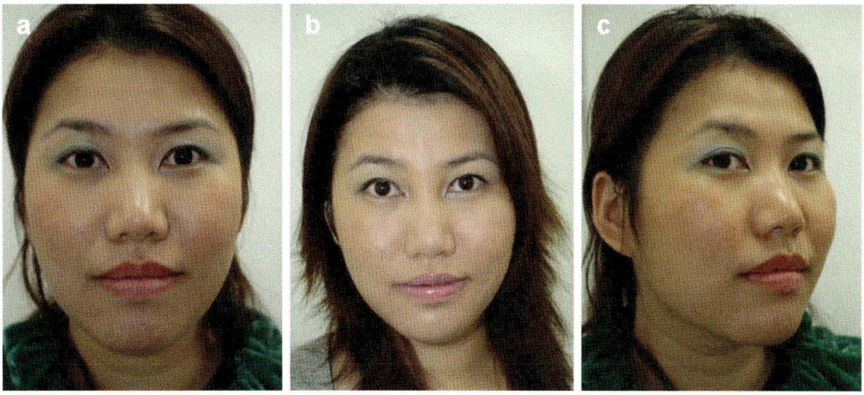

Fig. 4.66 Patient KH aged 25 presented with a "moon face" and wanted a "melon seed" contour. (**a**, **c**, **e**) Before. (**b**, **d**, **f**) Post-operative (age 27). Recontouring volume 26 ml (*Adapted from Ho* [17])

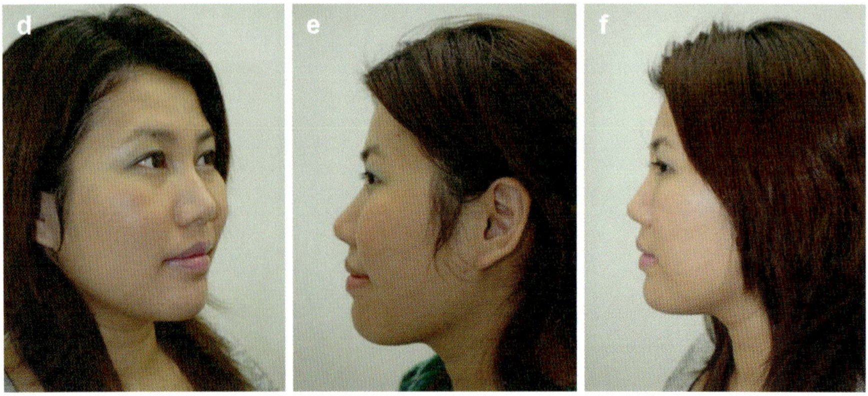

Fig. 4.66 (continued)

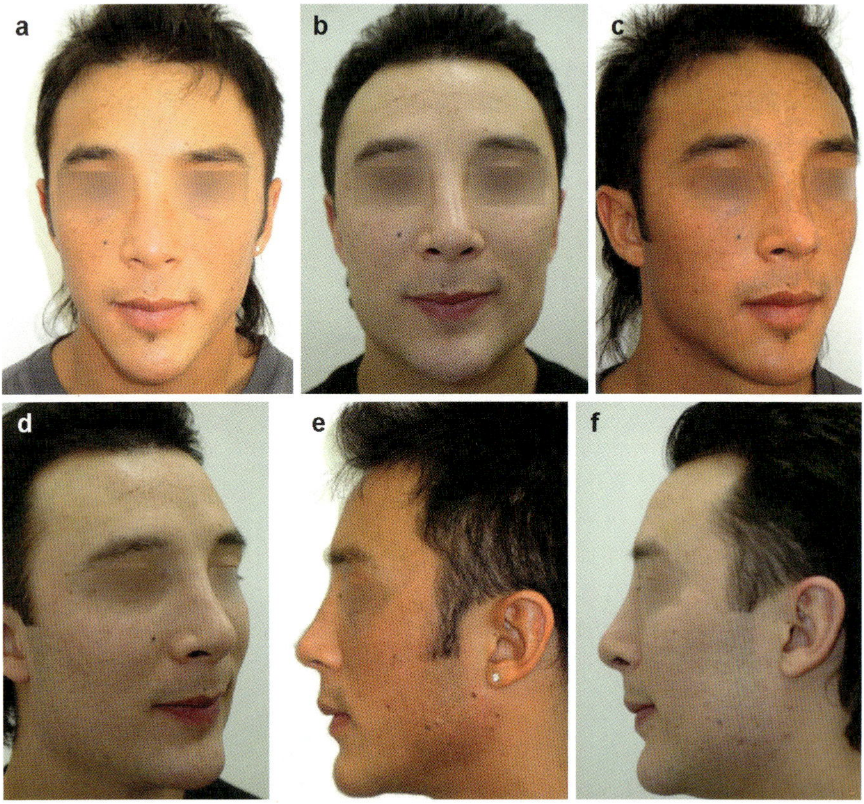

Fig. 4.67 Patient AG aged 24 disliked his triangular face and pointed chin; wanted a stronger lower jaw and rectangular face. (**a**, **c**, **e**) Before. (**b**, **d**, **f**) Post-operative aged 27. Recontouring volume 163 ml (*Adapted from Ho* [17])

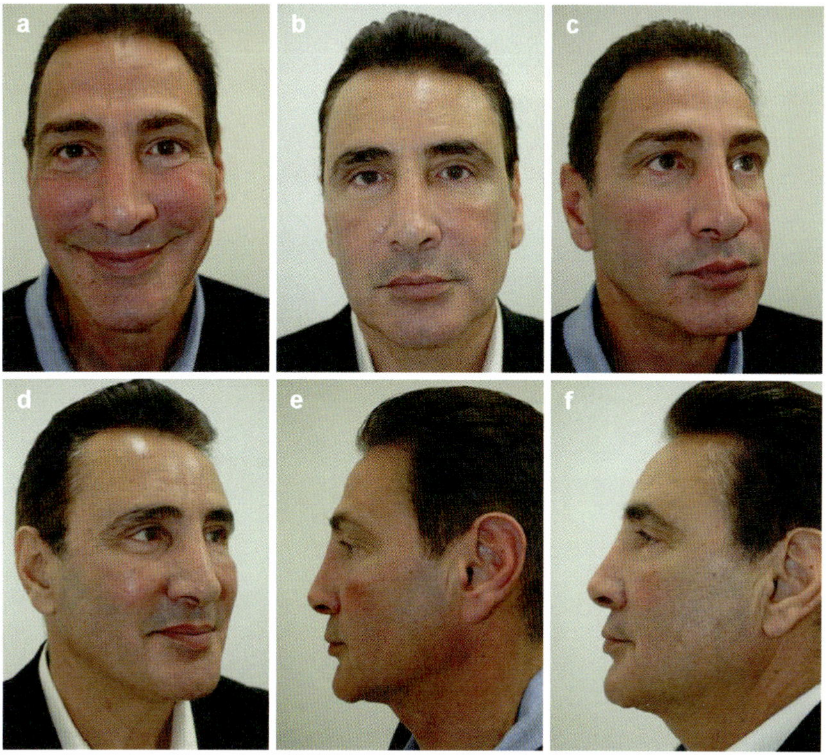

Fig. 4.68 Patient JA aged 53 years wanted his narrow face widened. (**a**, **c**, **e**) Before. (**b**, **d**, **f**) Post-operative aged 55. Recontouring volume was 210 ml (*Adapted from Ho* [17])

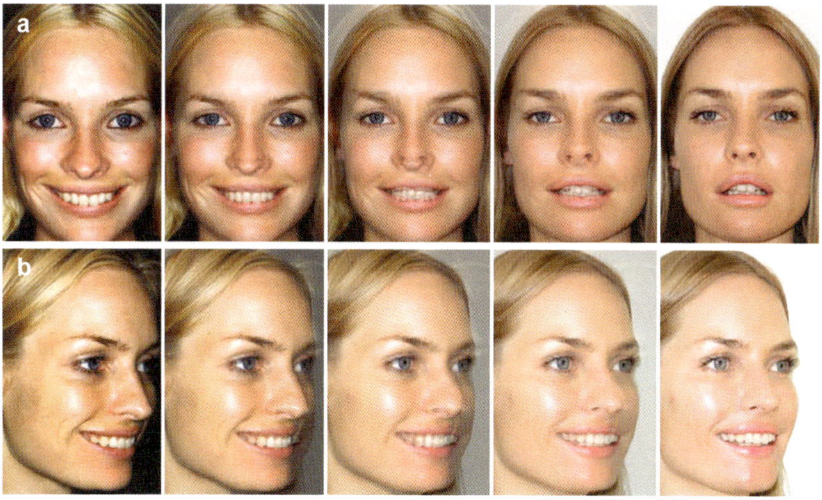

Fig. 4.69 (**a–c**) Patient LJ smiling. First facial optimisation patient (1999); Sequence morphing series from 2 years post-operative (2001) to 8 years post-operative (2009) in three views. Recontouring volume 105 ml. (**d–f**) Patient LJ face at rest. Sequence morphing series from 2 years post-operative (2001) to 9 years post-operative (2009) in three views

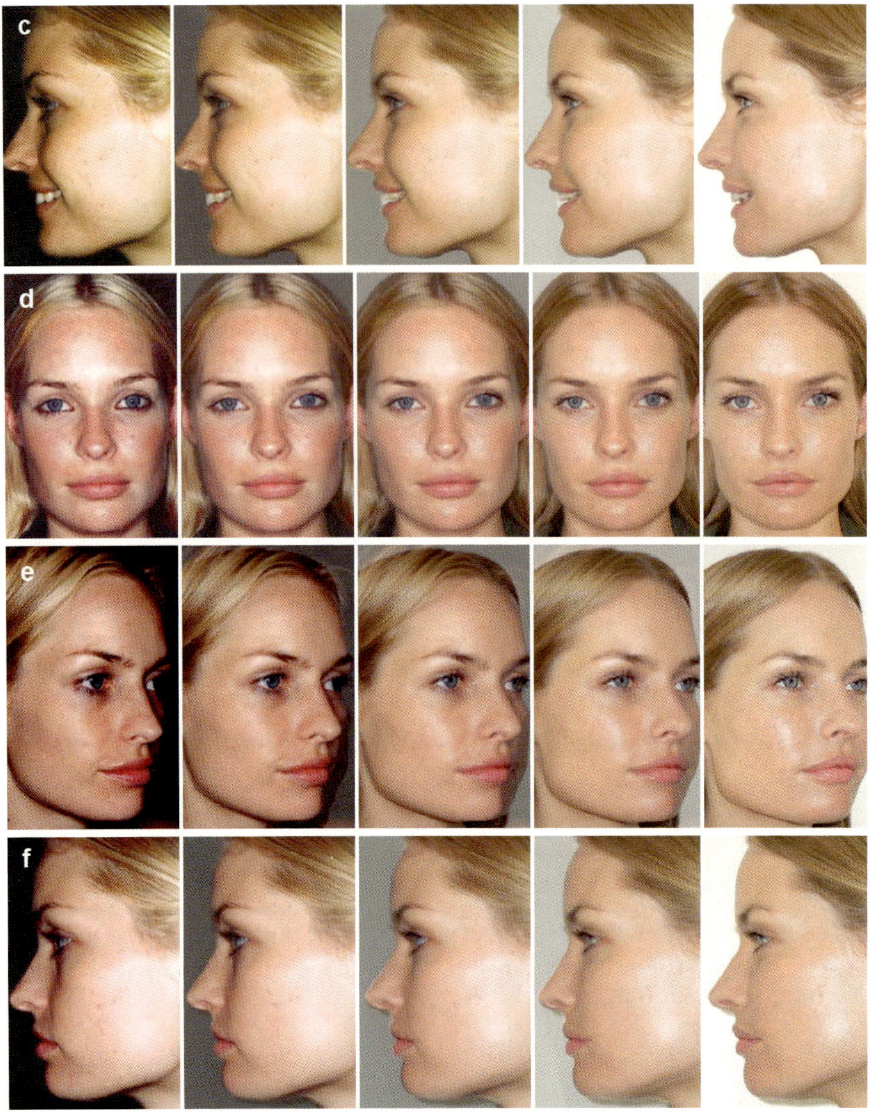

Fig. 4.69 (continued)

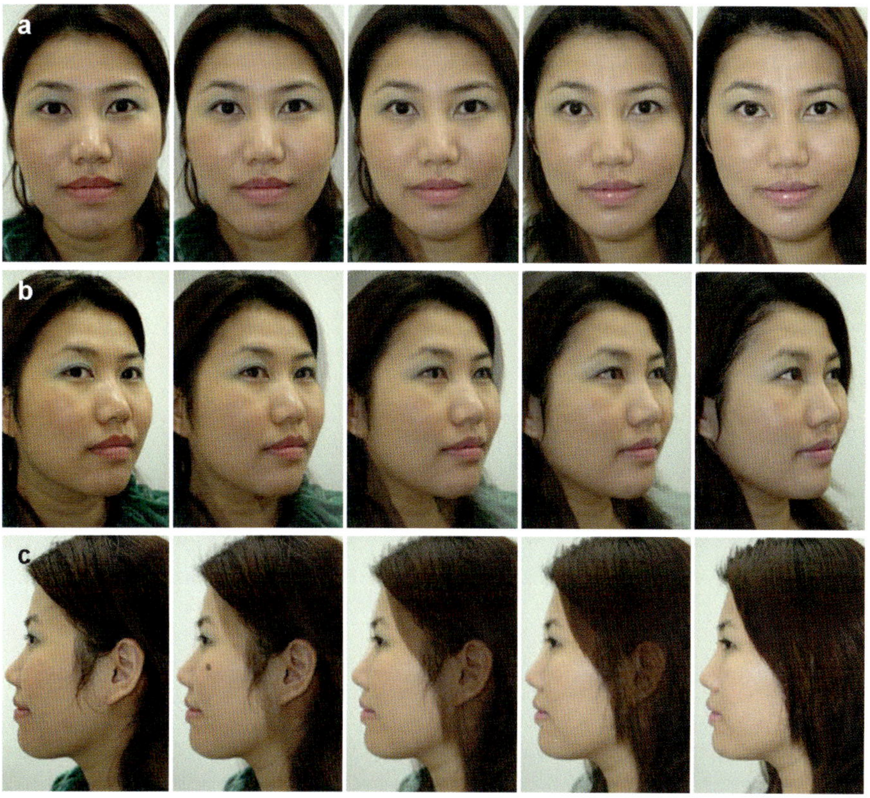

Fig. 4.70 (**a**–**c**) Patient KH. Sequence morphing in three views from preoperative to 2 years postoperative. Recontouring volume 26 ml (Video 4.10)

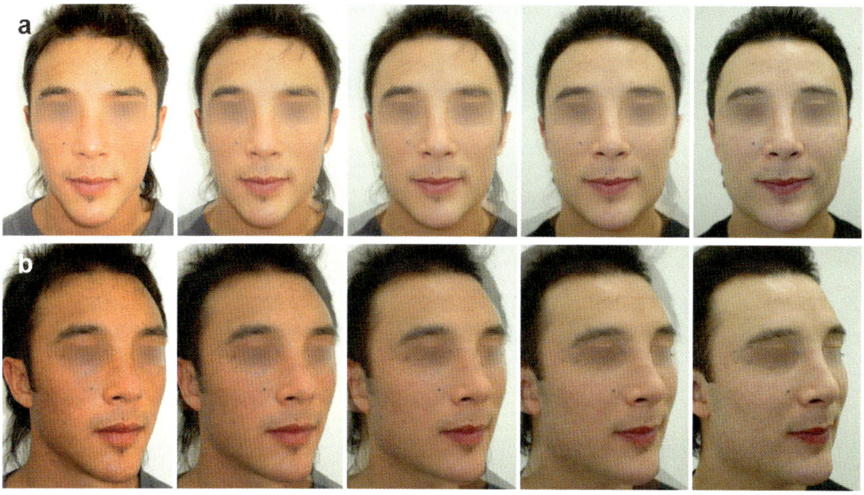

Fig. 4.71 (**a**–**c**) Patient AG. Sequence morphing in three views from preoperative to 3 years postoperative. Recontouring volume 163 ml

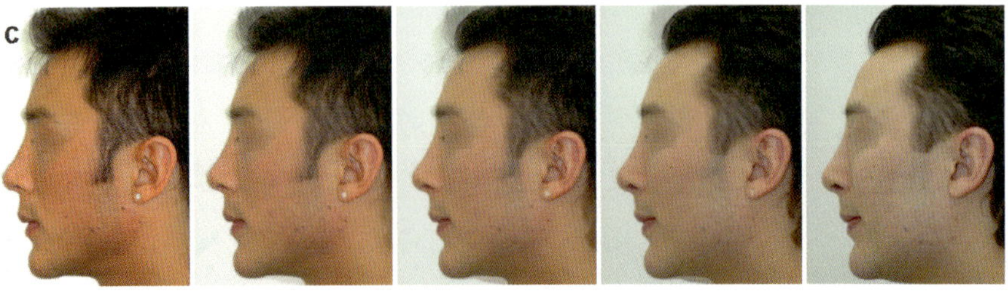

Fig. 4.71 (continued)

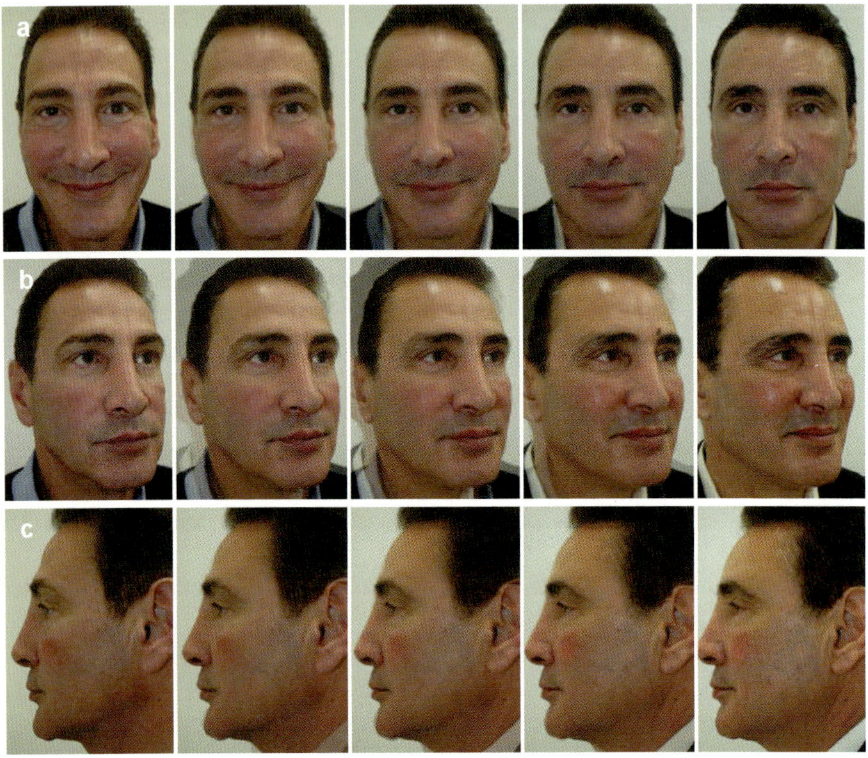

Fig. 4.72 (**a**–**c**) Patient JA. Sequence morphing from preoperative to 2 years post-operative. Recontouring volume 210 ml

Cheek Construction

Selective injection across the plane changeover junction to above junction ipsilateral ear and side of the head. (Cheek contour enforcement loop design takes in lateral tail extension.)

Oriental Cheek

Oriental cheek is a short tapered, "bottom" heavy wedge with a short flat "tail".

Lateral cheek pilaster sharply curved and inclined—generates broad appearance.

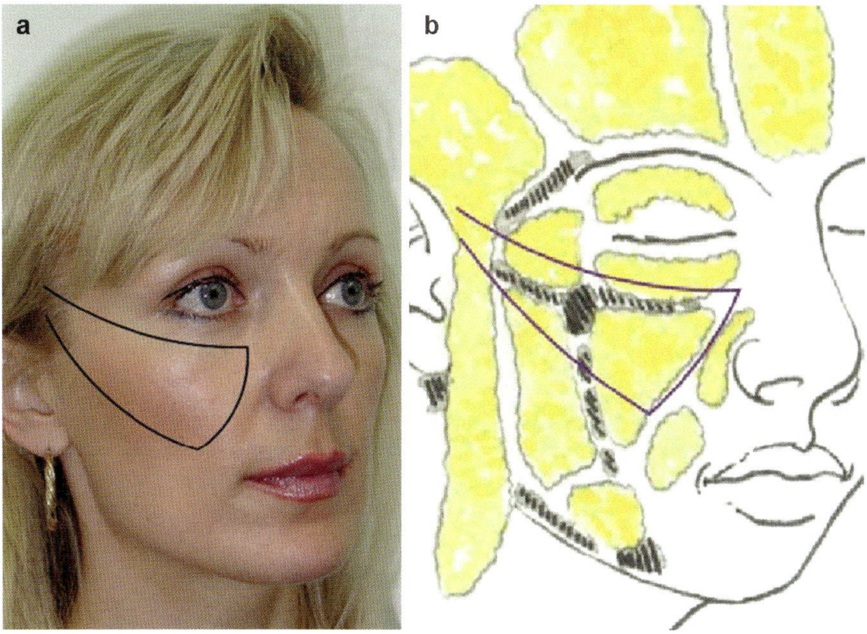

Fig. 4.73 (**a**, **b**) Cheek is biplane and straddles five fat compartments

Appearance of the old flat occidental cheek with heavy nasolabial folds.

Optimal construction—selectively targeted injection to the upper lateral quadrant cheek and around corner obliquely to ear-head junction.

Overly bulky nasolabial region is reduced by precise liposuction. (Occidentalisation of oriental cheek.)

Patient KH in Fig. 4.70a–c cheek construction lacked finesse (inadequately tapered).

Lower Jaw

Incline of the ramus pilaster (and width of mentum) determines the width of the face.

Narrow Lower Jaw Correction (Widen Lower Jaw)

Volumise mandibular angle to lower (selective microinjection in superficial planes for tenting effect).

Inject volume to lower vertical and proximal oblique limbs of ramus pilaster.

"Point" mentum—selective microinjection to medial third mental pilasters.

Lower mentum—selective micro of lower edge mentum.

Square Jaw Correction

Lipo-reduce mandibular angle, its lower border.

Lower mentum—selective micro injection of lower border of mental pilasters.

Correction of the Long Languid Face
Correction reverses procedure of patient in Figs. 4.66a–f and 4.70a–c (“moon face” to “melon seed”).

Lateral cheek pilaster realigned more obliquely by selective appropriate volumising upper medial quadrant cheek wedge.

Increase volume lower half of orbital—temporal—zygomatic pilaster.

Augment mandibular angles.

Pre-procedure Pilaster Markings (Fig. 4.74a, b)
Essential in planning—on photos in two views or use Keynote app with print out.

Preoperative markings on patient face; proposed new pilasters.

4.5 Global Panorama

“Physiologically ageing is largely due to progressive attenuation of blood supply to the tissues. Therefore, iatrogenic de-vascularisation from multiplane dissection is potentially deleterious to the face. The other problem challenging patients and their surgeon is the potential of producing rejuvenation that is unnatural appearance [3] and in some cases accompanied by deformity of the facial contours and face/neck interphase and ear. Poor or mismanagement of the SMAS in face-lift surgery often leads to

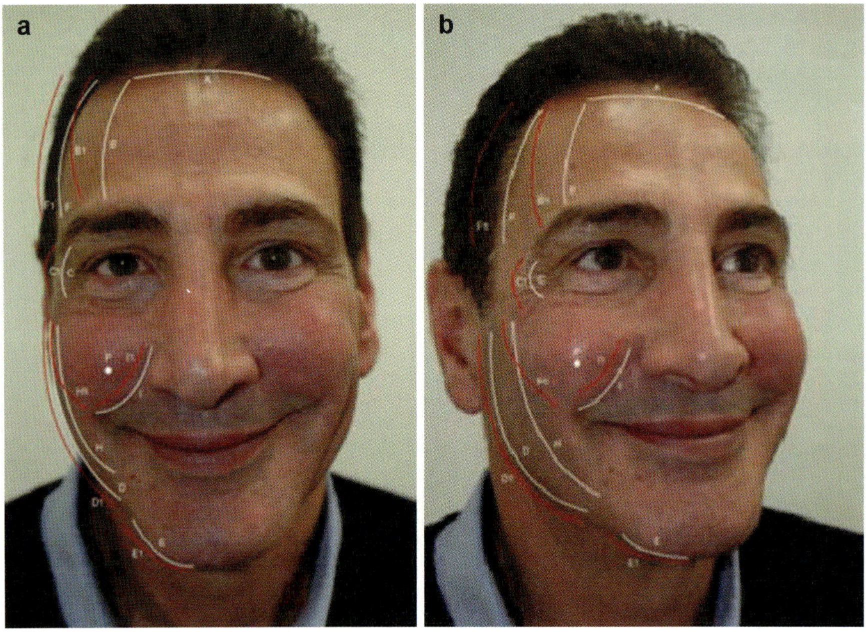

Fig. 4.74 (**a**, **b**) Planned preoperative markings on photographs; existing pilasters in white and proposed new pilasters in red

a broad appearance of the lower face post-operatively [3] as the large poorly supported mid-portion of the SMAS lies at the changeover junction of the front and lateral planes of the face. Lifting facial skin and suturing it under tension to the preauricular skin edge often lead to malrotation and distortion of the ear and earlobe. The described congruent face-lift addresses the three-dimensional structure of the face and avoids deformation at the front side changeover junction and face/neck interphase".

4.5.1 Ostium Eingang

Face-lifting began at the turn of the of the twentieth century on both sides of the Atlantic with timid conservative incision excision/closure of the skin in front of the ear running into the lower temple and below and behind the earlobe. A curved incision was used, and this progressed rapidly to wide subcutaneous undermining and suture closure with a dorsal cephalic vector with predictable broadening of the lower face. This 2D based dorsal cephalic vector has stubbornly remained the popular norm to this day.

The one exception was Joseph of Berlin who used a vertical preauricular incision extending into the temple with a "front cut" and wide undermining. A sole cephalic vector in the lateral plane provided three and half cm lift. This engineered a smooth trim face, submentum and neck! He had observed the obvious—a large loose sling in the lower face and neck—and intuitively deduced correctly (like Hollander's aristocrat patient) that "sling" tightening would tighten and smooth the "sling" and "un-telescope" the crumpled neck sleeve. This witnessed the birth of the effective side plane vertical vector elevation in 1911 which was unfortunately consigned to the dustbin of history for a hundred years!

4.5.2 Digression

Non-surgical Face-Lift
Sulamanidze's APTOS thread lift [22] is minimally invasive and unlikely to be classified as a surgical operation, but it merits attention; the vectors designed are congruently placed respecting plane and sub-plane changeover junctions. The improvement though slight is natural-looking. It is the first procedure designed expressly to "cone" and elevate the cheek in the front plane!

Two-Dimensional Shortcomings
A problem challenging patients and their surgeon working on a two-dimensional platform is the potential to produce rejuvenation that is unnatural in appearance [3] and in some cases accompanied by deformity of facial contours, neck and face/neck interphase.

Lifting facial skin and suturing it under tension to the preauricular skin edge may cause long-term malrotation of the ear and distraction distortion of its lobe.

Anterior cervical plasties described over the past decades involving excision of anterior borders, division of the bands horizontally at the upper level of the thyroid cartilage and suture of the decussation lead to an unnaturally looking neck. Gianpappa and Hoefflin using strong sutures from mastoid tip to mastoid tip to attain a better neck definition [10–12] compounded this with a "garrotted appearance".

Physiological Compromises
Physiologically, ageing is due largely to progressive attenuation of blood supply to the tissues. Iatrogenic de-vascularisation from extensive multiplane dissection is unphysiological.

Useful Innovations
De-epithelialised short dermal pennant flaps (Fig. 4.27a, b) designed and carried out in the preauricular skin (thrown away in all face-lifts) are anchored by suture fixation to the mastoid and temporal fascia; this allows tension-free closure of the lateral cheek skin flap away from the vulnerable ear.

Trans-cartilaginous horizontal mattress sutures give a strong closure and produce neat preauricular scars.

Towards a Rational Approach
Early work towards the end of the last century with fat micro graft volume-expansion rejuvenation technique (rejuvenative facial lipomorphoplasty) gave an insight into the three-dimensional structure of the face with their spatial transition zone highlights and parameters. Success with restoration of structural volume deficit in facial rejuvenation gave an insight into the probable anatomical structure and support system of the mid- and lower face which made this and facial optimisation successful.

4.5.3 Principalisation

Three-Dimensional Platform
The face (or head) is a three-dimensional anatomical structure with a front plane, two side planes and two horizontal planes. These are margined by changeover junctions (pilasters) which are distinct, convex and highly reflective. The front/side change over pilaster is 80–85°; much of the lower half of the lateral plane is visible as a rhomboid and is very prominent in some faces. Flattening the contour of this pilaster widens the appearance of the face. The face (/head) continues downwards onto the cylindrical neck; the anterior half of the face protrudes beyond the cephalic end of the neck cylinder with a concavely contoured interphase.

Support System of Mid- and Lower Face
This consists of a twin suspension system of ligaments/septa and "walled in "structural volume" competent soft tissue/fat compartments mutually holding up well the

mid- and lower face in the young. The whole is suspended by a top horizontal curtain rod and a lower "lead weight/curtain rod" with a curved oblique "staying system" at the front/side plane changeover junction. This is quintessential in surgical rejuvenation as its transition zone is not rigid.

Ageing
The ageing process imposes a continuous changing dynamic pattern as a result of ligament/septa attenuation/lengthening and compartment de-voluming; at times, these two processes do not proceed in tandem (Video 4.11 - Aging face/neck).

Biomechanical Intervention
Vector and contour congruent enforcement loops are used to recontour, recompress and securely fix the ptotic out of shaped facial compartments (features) to the elevated youthful latitude (Video 4.12 - Reverse aging face/neck).

Re-voluming the de-volumed face with little skin excess and ptosis restores adequate structural volume to reverse the dynamic ageing pattern where ligament/septa strength and length are slightly compromised.

Aesthetic recruitment of adjacent compartment's subunits is used to reconstruct the size, shape, position and angle of relevant pilasters to engineer a suitable change in the size, shape, disposition and arrangement of the facial planes and sub-planes to optimise the appearance of the face.

4.5.4 Exitus Ausfahrt

This work introduces a three-dimensional platform together with an integrated support system for the lower face, neck and their interphase.

The three-dimensional platform defines facial planes, sub-planes and their changeover junctions which are border highlights or pilasters which denote real-time spatial transition. It provides a rational template for design of face-lift and other rejuvenation procedures.

The integrated three-dimensional support consists of a tight (in the young) suspension system of ligaments/septa and structural volume competent compartments of soft tissue and fat "walled in" by this ligament/septa suspension system mutually holding up the free-hanging mid- and lower face "sandwich".

Facial rejuvenation techniques must work within the parameters imposed by the three-dimensional structure and the integrated support system for the lower face, neck and their interphase.

(The L Ho needle which made easy vertical front planed cheek "coning" and elevation via oblique side plane transit and anchoring was developed in 2005, almost a hundred years after the Joseph 3.5 cm side plane vertical elevation.)

References

1. Alghoul M, Codner MA (2013) Retaining ligaments of the face. Review of anatomy and clinical applications. Aesthet Surg J 405:1–14
2. Mendelson BC (1997) SMAS fixation to the facial skeleton: rationale and results. Plast Reconstr Surg 100:1834–1842
3. Jackson I, Yavuzer R, Beale B (2000) Simultaneous facelift & carbon dioxide laser resurfacing: a safe technique? Aesthetic Plast Surg 24(1):1–10
4. Joseph J (1931) Nasenplastik und sonstige Gesichsplastik nebst einem anhang uber mammaplastik. Verlag von Curt Kabitzsch, Leipzig
5. Lexer, E; Die gesamte Wiederherstellungschirurgie (Leipzig, Barth), Zugleich 2, Auflage der Wiederherstellungschirurgie, Mit 1910 Abbidungen im Text, Band 11, 1931.
6. Saylan Z (1999) The S-lift. Less is more. Aesth Surg Jour 19(5):406–409
7. Saylan Z (2002) Purse-string-formed plication of SMAS with zygomatic bone fixation. Plast Reconstr Surg 110(2):667–671
8. Tonnard PL, Verpaele A, Monstrey S, Van Landuyt K, Blondeel P, Hamdi M, Matton G (2002) Minimal access cranial suspension lift: a modified S lift. Plast Reconstr Surg 109(6):2074–2086
9. Tonnard PL, Verpaele A, Gaia S (2005) Optimising results from minimal access cranial suspension lifting (MACS-lift). Aesthetic Plast Surg 29(4):213–220
10. Hoefflin SM (1998) The extended supraplatysmal plane (ESP) face lift. Plast Reconstr Surg 101:494–503
11. Gianpapa V, Di Bernado BE (1995) Neck recontouring with suture suspension and liposuction: an alternative for early rhytidectomy candidate. Aesthetic Plast Surg 19(3):217–233
12. Gianpappa V, Bitzos I, Ramirez O, Granick M (2005) Long term results of suture suspension platysmaplasty for neck rejuvenation: a 13 year follow-up evaluation. Aesthetic Plast Surg 29(5):332–340
13. Cronin TD, Biggs TM (1971) The T-Z-plasty for the male 'Turkey Gobbler' neck. Plast Reconstr Surg 47(6):534–538
14. Adamson JE, Toksu AE (1981) Progress in rhytidectomy by platysma-SMAS rotation and elevation. Plast Reconstr Surg 68(1):23–33
15. Guerrero-Santos J, Espaillat L, Morales F (1974) Muscular lift in cervical rhytidectomy. Plast Reconstr Surg 54(2):127–131
16. Ho LCY (2002) Refinements in rejuvenative facial lipomorphoplasty. Aesthetic Plast Surg 26(5):329–334
17. Ho LCY (2011) Facial optimisation. Chin J Aesthetic Plast Surg 11:702–708
18. Ho LCY (2012) Contour and vector congruent facelift. Chin J Aesthetic Plast Surg 11:702–704
19. Ho LCY, Yin Z, Fan J (2014) Visuality. Chin J Aesthetic Plast Surg 9:573–576
20. Gregory RL (1997) Eye and brain: the psychology of seeing, 5th edn. Princeton University Press, Princeton, NJ
21. Chang L, Tsao D (2017) The code for facial identity in the primate brain. Cell 169(6):1013–1028
22. Sulamanidze MA, Shiffman MA, Paikidze TG, Sulamanidze GM, Gavasheli LG (2001) Facial lifting with APTOS threads. Int J Cosmet Surg Aesthetic Dermatol 3:275–281

Index

L.C.Y. Ho et al., *The Congruent Facelift*,
https://doi.org/10.1007/978-3-319-69090-2

Printed by Printforce, the Netherlands